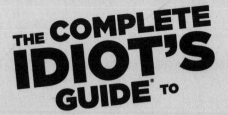

Plant-Based
Nutrition

by Julieanna Hever, M.S., R.D., C.P.T.

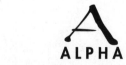

ALPHA

A member of Penguin Group (USA) Inc.

ALPHA BOOKS

Published by the Penguin Group

Penguin Group (USA) Inc., 375 Hudson Street, New York, New York 10014, USA

Penguin Group (Canada), 90 Eglinton Avenue East, Suite 700, Toronto, Ontario M4P 2Y3, Canada (a division of Pearson Penguin Canada Inc.)

Penguin Books Ltd., 80 Strand, London WC2R 0RL, England

Penguin Ireland, 25 St. Stephen's Green, Dublin 2, Ireland (a division of Penguin Books Ltd.)

Penguin Group (Australia), 250 Camberwell Road, Camberwell, Victoria 3124, Australia (a division of Pearson Australia Group Pty. Ltd.)

Penguin Books India Pvt. Ltd., 11 Community Centre, Panchsheel Park, New Delhi—110 017, India

Penguin Group (NZ), 67 Apollo Drive, Rosedale, North Shore, Auckland 1311, New Zealand (a division of Pearson New Zealand Ltd.)

Penguin Books (South Africa) (Pty.) Ltd., 24 Sturdee Avenue, Rosebank, Johannesburg 2196, South Africa

Penguin Books Ltd., Registered Offices: 80 Strand, London WC2R 0RL, England

Copyright © 2011 by Julieanna Hever

THE COMPLETE IDIOT'S GUIDE TO and Design are registered trademarks of Penguin Group (USA) Inc.

International Standard Book Number: 978-1-61564-101-7
Library of Congress Catalog Card Number: 2011901230

13 12 11   8 7 6 5

Interpretation of the printing code: The rightmost number of the first series of numbers is the year of the book's printing; the rightmost number of the second series of numbers is the number of the book's printing. For example, a printing code of 11-1 shows that the first printing occurred in 2011.

Printed in the United States of America

Most Alpha books are available at special quantity discounts for bulk purchases for sales promotions, premiums, fund-raising, or educational use. Special books, or book excerpts, can also be created to fit specific needs.

For details, write: Special Markets, Alpha Books, 375 Hudson Street, New York, NY 10014.

Publisher: *Marie Butler-Knight*
Associate Publisher: *Mike Sanders*
Executive Managing Editor: *Billy Fields*
Acquisitions Editor: *Tom Stevens*
Senior Development Editor: *Christy Wagner*
Senior Production Editor: *Kayla Dugger*

Copy Editor: *Krista Hansing Editorial Services, Inc.*
Cover Designer: *Rebecca Batchelor*
Book Designers: *William Thomas, Rebecca Batchelor*
Indexer: *Johnna VanHoose Dinse*
Layout: *Brian Massey*
Senior Proofreader: *Laura Caddell*

This book is dedicated to my plant-strong rock, Aviv, and our precious little plantlings, Maya and Benny.

"Julieanna Hever shares the very best of health and nutrition in this wonderful new book. *The Complete Idiot's Guide to Plant-Based Nutrition* is the perfect plan for getting your diet in gear. Whether you've wanted to slim down, improve your energy, lower your cholesterol, improve diabetes, or just look great in the mirror, Julieanna shows you how remarkably easy it is to get there. She also demystifies the world of nutrition. If you are asking about where you'll find protein, which foods are the most vitamin-rich, or what supplements you might need, you'll have Julieanna Hever's in-depth knowledge with you every step of the way. It's like having your own personal plant-based dietitian right there with you as you shop and cook. This immensely practical book will be your trusted resource."

—Neal D. Barnard, M.D., Adjunct Associate Professor of Medicine, George Washington University School of Medicine, and President, Physicians Committee for Responsible Medicine

Contents

Foreword

A new world of food and its effects on health is now upon us. Eating whole, plant-based foods is the wave of the future if we have any chance of improving our health, reducing health-care costs, stemming the tide of environmental assaults, and creating a less violent and more peaceful world. It begins with our understanding of food and then using it properly.

The scientific evidence is now convincing, and a growing number of people are becoming aware of how beneficial really good food can be. As a life-long researcher, I lecture far and wide about the scientific evidence that underlies this kind of food, and I am impressed with the number of people who find this information so compelling. It is my experience that people very much want to be healthy and, further, that they are much more interested in the relationship between food and health than many professionals are willing to acknowledge. The two most frequent questions asked of me are *Why have we not known this information before?* and *How do I prepare the food?* But to get such a dialogue started, it is important to start with a discussion of what kind of nutritional effects might be expected from the consumption of whole, plant-based foods.

We need a book that sets the stage for this discussion, one that does not require enrollment in serious courses on the complex biology of nutrition. Here is a great place to start. Julieanna Hever is a professionally trained dietitian, a public lecturer on the subject, and now is ideally placed to write a nutrition book for the general public. Unlike most nutrition books, from the simplest to the most erudite, which are focused too much, either directly or indirectly, on what individual nutrients do or don't do, this book is focused on the exceptional health value of *whole*, plant-based foods, with little or no added fat, sugar, or salt.

As an aside, I should mention that, during my lectures, one of the most frequent questions I am asked is how much fat and oil can or should be added to food. My best guess is none. First, food can be made tasty without smothering it with fat—people like fat and become addicted to it—and second, without this added fat (as used in fried foods, in baked goods, and in salad dressings), we can discover new, health-generating tastes that were previously suppressed. If and when we give this idea a try, we will be pleasantly surprised and pleased with the health benefits that will come our way.

I recommend this book as a starter to set you on your path to a healthier future. Start your new dietary lifestyle with this book. You can't go wrong. When you begin to personally experience the benefits, I predict that you will be sharing copies with friends and family.

T. Colin Campbell, Ph.D.
Co-author, *The China Study*
Professor Emeritus of Nutrition, Cornell University

Introduction

For the first time in history, we are overfed and undernourished. Health care is a disaster, where we lose billions of dollars a year supporting disease symptom management. People are sicker and fatter than ever before, and ironically, we have the most access to healthful food and medical care. Although the reasons surrounding these issues may be complex, the solution is simple. It all comes down to the food on your plate.

Eating healthfully may very well be the most confusing and frustrating part of everyday life. Frequent fads and trends come and go, leaving you lost in their wake, uncertain about the failed promises of successfully achieving perfect health and ideal weight. Distinguishing between fact and fiction is virtually impossible with the never-ending onslaught of hype in television, on the Internet, in magazines, in books, and through word-of-mouth. Anyone can consider himself an expert, but what is he really trying to sell? Food policy has become entirely politicized. Thus, our nutrition guidelines come indirectly from food manufacturers, not the most objective resource for information.

Physicians receive minimal, if any, nutrition education in medical school, yet they're the front-line people providing guidance and care. Western medicine has become a game of identifying a symptom and applying a remedy for that symptom (a.k.a. chronic disease management). Never before have drug manufacturers sold their prescription medications directly to the consumer as they do now. Television commercials alternate between ads for fast food, junk food, and a new medication to help alleviate your symptoms from consuming those products.

It's time to see the forest instead of the trees. Health is not merely the absence of disease, nor are symptoms of poor health to be medicated and ignored. Instead, it's time to redefine health and nutrition.

Fortunately, a movement is well underway, confirming that what you eat can and does prevent, and even reverse, chronic disease. Researchers, physicians, and dietitians including myself have witnessed multitudes of people regain true health, ridding their dependence on medications and addictive foods. You can change your future and be responsible for how you look and feel simply by making the right food choices.

Whether this is your first foray into the plant-based world or you're a well-seasoned veteran, a plethora of facts and tips readily await you in the following chapters. Proceed through the pages to discover the most current advances in health and nutrition while you build your nutritional database and reap the rewards.

Everything you need to know to achieve optimal health is in your hands right now. Welcome to the gorgeously exciting and health-creating plant-based world!

How This Book Is Organized

This book is divided into four parts, each representing distinct attributes of plant-based nutrition:

Part 1, The Benefits of a Plant-Based Diet, offers a comprehensive course in nutrition fundamentals, dissecting what your food consists of. This part explains what your body requires for optimal health and where to get those nutrients. Get ready for the hot-off-the-presses Plant-Based Food Guide Pyramid, which will redefine what you've previously experienced and give you a new set of food groups to feast your hungry eyes upon.

Part 2, Living a Plant-Based Life, debunks most of the nutritional misinformation we've been fed over the years. It offers an entirely new perspective on weight loss and clarifies the most commonly confused health information. Take a stroll down the aisles of the supermarket with a plant-based eye, and you'll discover a whole-istic approach to food shopping. Learn how and why you need to incorporate a fitness program into your schedule to achieve optimum health, and see how much more fabulous you'll feel after you've done so. Finally, get answers to your supplement concerns so you can put to rest the notion that good health equals taking the right pills.

Part 3, Special Considerations, is dedicated to everyone who has been a baby, had a baby, raised a child, succeeded in athletics, battled the bulge, and/or confronted illness. Throughout your lifespan, your health needs change. This part breaks down all the nutrition concerns that come up in different situations, providing guidance so you can take the reins and control your destiny.

Armed with all the knowledge you've gained about what you need to do to thrive in your body, **Part 4, The Plant-Based Recipe Box,** shows you exactly how to do so. Master the art of dining out, stocking your kitchen, and nutrifying recipes to meet the guidelines described in this book. Then indulge your taste buds with whole-food recipes—more than 45 of them!—you can easily prepare and share as you learn tips to maximize your time in the kitchen, regardless of your expertise.

In the appendixes, you'll find a glossary of terms, a week's worth of sample meal plans, Dietary Reference Intake charts, and a list of handy resources for you to continue your plant-based journey.

Extras

Throughout the book, you'll find sidebars to guide you and offer additional information. Here's what to look for:

DEFINITION

These sidebars clarify jargon and other questionable terms.

MIXED GREENS

Miscellaneous thoughts and additives fill these sidebars.

HEALTHY HINT

These facts and tips increase your knowledge and help put the concepts into action.

PLANT PITFALL

These sidebars feature warnings and cautionary advice you should check out.

Acknowledgments

I'd love to offer gratitude to several people. For giving me the opportunity to write this book, I offer a huge thank you to Marilyn Allen, for believing in me right from the start; Tom Stevens, for this wonderful opportunity; Brenda Davis, my mentor, role model, and idol; and my brilliant editor, Shelly Vaughan James, who transformed my green writing with her straight-forward fabulousness. Thank you to Christy Wagner, Kayla Dugger, and Krista Hansing at Alpha Books for your amazing work and support.

To my heroes, whose pioneering spirits are literally changing the world. My deepest gratitude to Dr. T. Colin Campbell, the "Father of Modern Nutrition," for all his advice, support, inspiration, and absolute genius (and for writing the foreword to this book). Deep gratitude to John Robbins, the match who sparked my flame and whose wisdom continues to fuel my fire to want to do better. Thank you to the unstoppable Dr. Joel Fuhrman, for generously offering his advice and guidance. Sincere thanks to the courageous and world-beautifying Dr. Neal Barnard, for his immediate assistance on any matter. Thanks to Dr. John McDougall, for his persistence, passion, and certainty. Much appreciation to Ginny Messina, for her precision and clarity. And to my dearly loved, beautiful, and talented friend and colleague Dina Aronson, for her ceaseless support, making me laugh when I needed it most, reminding me of the big picture, and for performing the nutrient analyses for the recipes in this book.

Special thanks to my culinary mastermind and dear friend, Beverly Lynn Bennett, who has provided me a glimpse of virtuosity-in-motion. And to my dear Chef AJ, for her delicious contributions to the recipe section and for inspiring me in my kitchen. Much appreciation to Sherri Nestorowich for bringing my food guide pyramid to life and to PCRM for sharing their Power Plate. Thank you to the clever and awesome Zel Allen, for her amazing salad and emergency dressing consult. Thank you to Kappel LeRoy Clarke, the guru of conditioning and movement, who endlessly sparks my creativity; and my beloved Broccolini, Jesse Pomeroy, for his eternal support and ingenious talent.

On a personal note, words cannot express how much appreciation I want to offer my family. My mom, my biggest fan, who always knew this book was coming and tells me daily I can succeed at anything I want to in life. My ema, who inspires me to be a better person. My dad, for all his advice and tough love. My sweet sister, Rachel, for rescuing me when I needed her. Thank you to my fabulous family for your love and patience. And most of all, to my angelic little plantlings, Maya and Benny, may you continue to sprout beautifully and brilliantly as you've done thus far. And to the love of my life, Aviv, thank you for being my plant-strong rock … I am eternally grateful.

Trademarks

All terms mentioned in this book that are known to be or are suspected of being trademarks or service marks have been appropriately capitalized. Alpha Books and Penguin Group (USA) Inc. cannot attest to the accuracy of this information. Use of a term in this book should not be regarded as affecting the validity of any trademark or service mark.

The Benefits of a Plant-Based Diet

Part

1

More and more people are getting interested in plant-based nutrition as the numerous health benefits associated with this way of eating are coming to light. But what exactly constitutes a plant-based diet, and how do you go about exploring it for yourself? That's what Part 1 is all about. It explains how to eat a whole-food, plant-based diet so you can see how easy this health-promoting way of life is.

Stay tuned for a Nutrition 101 lesson filled with everything nature has to offer. In the following chapters, we explore what your food is made of, what your body thrives on, and how to merge the two. I also help you redefine your mind-set toward food and eating as you begin to switch from the confusing and irresponsible rules you've been taught your whole life to a new set of plant-based guidelines.

Find the beauty in your plate and on your palate with whole-plant foods, and see how your life grows more colorful as you incorporate the ideas into daily practice!

What Plant-Based Nutrition Is All About

In This Chapter

- A closer look at plant-based eating
- Comparing a plant-based diet and other veg diets
- Healthy versus unhealthy veg diets
- What plant-based eating can do for you

Eating a plant-based diet is nothing new. People have been doing it for years, under the titles "vegetarian" and "vegan," among others. But don't let those "veg" titles scare you off. Getting your nutrition from plant-based foods is one of the best things you can do for your body and your well-being. And it's easier than you might think!

More and more people are realizing the benefits of plant-based nutrition. In response, restaurant menus are expanding to incorporate creative plant-based options, and even wholly plant-based restaurants are opening their doors. Supermarkets are carrying increasing amounts of plant products in every section, too. Health-care practitioners are also getting in on the action, exploring plant-based nutrition as a treatment for patients. Some of the most successful business moguls, politicians, and athletes have recently gone plant based, too. Even the U.S. Department of Agriculture (USDA) used the words *plant based* in its 2010 Dietary Guidelines.

Right now is the most electrifying and user-friendly time to be plant based! Get ready to be inspired by all the healthy advantages a plant-based diet offers!

What Is Plant Based?

Before we go any further, let's look at what "plant based" really means. *Plant based* simply means a way of eating based on foods that come from plants and avoiding animal products and highly processed foods. Simple enough, right? The addition of the words *whole food*, as in *whole-food, plant-based diet*, indicates the foods come directly from nature and have not been stripped of their original packaging.

PLANT PITFALL

Beware of junk food. Although some of it is technically plant based, eating a diet founded in non-nutritive foods such as white bread, potato chips, and diet cola isn't healthy and isn't the goal here. That's where the *whole-food* part of the diet comes in.

A whole-food, plant-based diet boasts a wide range of choices, including vegetables, fruits, whole grains, legumes, nuts, and seeds. Although these foods require very little processing and preparation, these earth-harvested ingredients can tempt your taste buds in dishes ranging from fine gourmet to casual comfort food.

Additionally, while studying populations, physicians and researchers have found that a whole-food, plant-based diet results in optimum health. The higher the percentage of the diet that comes from whole-plant foods, the lower the risk for heart disease, many cancers, type 2 diabetes, obesity, and autoimmune diseases. If you want to feel and look your best while savoring every bite, a whole-food, plant-based diet is the win-win option.

Vegan, Vegetarian, Plant Based

Now let's look at those other "veg" diets I mentioned earlier and see how they compare to a plant-based diet.

First up, *vegans*. Technically, a vegan is an herbivore, or plant eater, who lives solely on plant products and excludes all animal flesh, including that of poultry and fish, as well as any product made by an animal, such as milk and all other dairy products, eggs, gelatin, and honey. Typically, vegans don't wear clothing or other items made with animal products. That means no fur, leather, silk, wool, feathers, or pearls. They also avoid anything made with animal-based ingredients, such as some cosmetics, toiletries, or household goods.

A *vegetarian* doesn't eat animal flesh but may consume other animal-based foods like eggs and dairy. Vegetarianism has several subpopulations:

- Lacto-ovo vegetarians eat dairy (lacto) and eggs (ovo).

- Lacto-vegetarians eat dairy but not eggs.

- Ovo-vegetarians eat eggs but not dairy.

- Flexitarians (a contraction of the words *flexible* and *vegetarian*) eat mostly plant-based foods but occasionally eat meat, poultry, or fish, too.

- Semi-vegetarians exclude some meat (usually red meat) but still consume limited amounts of poultry, fish, and/or seafood.

DEFINITION

A **vegan** (*VEE-gan*) avoids consuming and using all animal products, including animal flesh, dairy, eggs, honey, leather, fur, silk, wool, and pearls. A **vegetarian** avoids eating meat, poultry, and fish. There are several types of vegetarianism.

When you think about it, although veganism and vegetarianism are plant-based diets for the most part, they're defined on what you *exclude* from your diet. Part of what makes a plant-based diet unique is that it defines the composition of what *is* included instead of what *isn't*.

The Health Benefits of a Plant-Based Diet

Over the last three or four decades, medical studies have led to discoveries that could potentially change the landscape of health care. Such studies have shown that eating a whole-food, plant-based diet can be key to proactive medical care.

Disease Prevention and Reversal

Diet has the power to prevent and reverse disease, according to pioneering physicians and researchers. They have documented patients who have regained their health, thanks in large part to diet. Their work has paved the path for future treatment protocols for chronic diseases.

T. Colin Campbell, Ph.D., author of *The China Study*, is one such researcher. A professor from Cornell University, Dr. Campbell has been able to debunk the myth that animal protein is healthy. In fact, his research shows animal protein to be a potent carcinogen, or cancer-causing agent. Furthermore, he has illustrated that a whole-food, plant-based diet is the most effective way to prevent and even reverse many cancers, heart disease, and the majority of other chronic diseases.

Dr. Campbell hypothesizes that we have only one disease process but many different expressions of that disease, depending on our genetic background. An elevated cholesterol level, now understood to be caused in part by animal protein, is a common factor among most chronic diseases.

We've spent the last several decades pointing to genetics as the primary source for which diseases you're likely to contract over your lifetime. Yet it's your lifestyle, especially what you eat, that establishes whether those genes are expressed and the illness flares up, or whether those harmful genes remain dormant. This means the food you choose to place on your plate has more control over your health than some predetermined destiny. In other words, your genes may load the gun, but your lifestyle pulls the trigger.

At the prestigious Cleveland Clinic, Dr. Caldwell Esselstyn reversed end-stage heart disease by using a whole-food, plant-based diet in a group of patients whose cardiologists basically sent them home to die. Dr. Dean Ornish, author of *Program for Reversing Heart Disease*, directed clinical research demonstrating the use of comprehensive lifestyle changes to undo severe coronary heart disease without drugs or surgery. Dr. John McDougall has reversed chronic disease for more than 30 years using a starch-centered diet. Dr. Joel Fuhrman uses a "Nutritarian" lifestyle—which is whole-food, plant-based—to heal his patients. Dr. Neal Barnard of Physician's Committee for Responsible Medicine (PCRM) has reversed type 2 diabetes with a whole-food, plant-based diet for years.

A clear connection has been established between diet and disease. It's time to put down the pills and potions and instead run to the nearest produce section!

Weight Management

Weight management has reached a critical impasse. After decades of searching for the perfect diet—from low-carb to grapefruit-intensive—the American population is only growing larger and more frustrated. Clearly, this approach has not been successful.

MIXED GREENS

More than two out of every three American adults are overweight or obese. As of 2008, approximately 72.5 million U.S. adults were categorized as obese, or 120 percent or more over their ideal body weight. Obesity is a contributing factor to many leading causes of death, including heart disease, stroke, diabetes, and some types of cancer.

Concentrating on a whole-food, plant-based diet is the most advantageous solution for achieving and sustaining optimum health and weight. In fact, several studies show that this type of eating plan does, indeed, produce the most favorable outcomes. And that's *without* any other changes in exercise or portion size! In other words, you can eat vegetables, fruits, whole grains, and legumes all you like and still achieve great weight-loss success.

Consuming large amounts of bulk with low energy density helps you feel fuller faster. That means incorporating large amounts of vegetables and fruits in your diet helps you maintain your ideal weight. And that's the idea behind the whole-food, plant-based diet.

Decreased Cholesterol Levels

High blood cholesterol has been associated with an increased risk of cardiovascular disease for decades. Factors that increase blood cholesterol levels include consuming foods that contain trans fatty acids (present only in processed foods), saturated fats, animal protein, and *dietary cholesterol* (found only in animal products).

DEFINITION

Dietary cholesterol is a waxy substance found in cell membranes and transported via the blood. An essential structural component of cell membranes, cholesterol is necessary for the manufacture of bile acids, steroid hormones, and fat-soluble vitamins, including vitamins A, D, E, and K.

Foods that improve cholesterol levels include fiber (found in all whole-plant foods exclusively) and omega-3 fatty acids (from flaxseeds, hempseeds, soybeans, and walnuts). Randomized controlled trials have confirmed that a whole-food, plant-based diet improves blood cholesterol levels.

Because high cholesterol is a common denominator in most chronic diseases, your profile can be considered an indicator for disease potential. For minimized risk, aim to keep your total cholesterol below 150 mg/dL, your LDL below 100 mg/dL, and your HDL above 45 mg/dL.

LDL stands for low-density lipoprotein and is the component of "bad" cholesterol. High levels of LDL in the blood contribute to the formation of plaque in your arteries, which leads to coronary artery disease. You want this number to remain low. On the contrary, HDL, or high-density lipoprotein, has the job of scooping bad cholesterol out of the blood and transporting it to the liver to be disposed of. Thus, a higher blood value of HDL is heart healthy. Ideally, try to achieve a ratio of two to one, LDL to HDL, for superior cardiovascular protection.

Improved Performance

Although the scientific data are not yet established, several world-class athletes partially credit a whole-food, plant-based diet with their improved athletic performance. From track and field to football, basketball, and body building, many superstars claim their enhanced success is due to following a plant-based diet.

Plant-based nutrition has become quite possibly the best medicine around. When compared to other ways of eating, whole-plant foods provide the most benefits in terms of achieving optimal health. If you combine all the current medications at your disposal, nothing comes close to the benefits of eating a whole-food, plant-based diet.

The Least You Need to Know

- Current research supports a whole-food, plant-based diet as the key to achieving optimum health.
- "Plant based" describes the types of foods included in a meal plan or any type of diet that's heavy on whole-plant foods.
- A whole-food, plant-based diet is the premier option for minimizing risk of disease, achieving optimum weight, and keeping cholesterol levels in check.

Breaking Down the Macronutrients

In This Chapter

- Energy-boosting carbs
- Plant-based protein powerhouses
- Fats and their functions

The colors, textures, aromas, and flavors of a delicious, freshly prepared meal all work together to stimulate your senses in anticipation of that first bite. Your mouth waters and your stomach grumbles as it eagerly looks forward to breaking down the macro- and micronutrients in every delicious morsel. Macronutrients are the calorie-providing nutrients your body requires in large amounts, including carbohydrates, protein, and fat. Micronutrients are required in small amounts and consist of the water- and fat-soluble vitamins, macrominerals, and trace elements.

In this chapter, I explain everything you need to know about the basics of macro-nutrition. (The micronutrients get their own chapter—Chapter 3.) So rev up your brain power and get ready for an essential lesson on nutrition!

Crazy About Carbs

Controversy over carbohydrates, or carbs, have continued to reign supreme in nutrition news for decades. Are they healthy, or are they fattening? Even the name itself has been mistakenly redefined to mean processed starchy foods. Let's take a look at the facts and make some sense of the carb craze.

Carbs are composed of carbon, hydrogen, and oxygen atoms, which make up the building blocks for a sugar, or saccharide, molecule. These molecules vary widely, from simple to complex, depending on how many saccharides are linked together. From sugars to fibers, carbs are an extremely important macronutrient that provides the vast majority of calories in your daily diet.

Carbs provide energy more quickly than any other fuel source and are the only type of energy the brain can utilize. When provided from whole sources such as vegetables, fruits, whole grains, and legumes, carbs come packaged with large amounts and varieties of vitamins, minerals, and phytochemicals.

You might have heard that carbs make you fat. That's a misunderstanding. Trendy, high-protein diets that promote eating animal products and processed foods filled with fat and refined sugars are what contribute to weight gain. But healthy, whole carbs have quite the opposite effect.

Simple Versus Complex Carbs

Simple is a term used to define carbohydrates made up of one or two sugar molecules, named *monosaccharides* and *disaccharides*, respectively.

Monosaccharides include glucose, fructose, and galactose, which are found in fruits, honey, and corn syrup. Edible disaccharides include sucrose (table sugar), lactose (milk sugar), and maltose. Disaccharides are found in cane and beet sugars, milk and milk products, and malt.

Polysaccharides, or complex carbohydrates, contain three or more sugars and can be divided into starch and fiber.

Starch, a complex form of sugars linked together, is digestible and provides an excellent source of energy. Plentiful in the plant kingdom, starch shows up primarily in seeds and roots. Food sources of starch include potatoes, wheat, maize, rice, barley, cassava, tapioca, rye, oats, and peas.

Resistant starch is a special type of starch that remains intact throughout the cooking process and during the enzyme breakdown of digestion. Therefore, it's actually a fiber. Resistant starch helps control blood sugar, lowers blood cholesterol and triglyceride concentrations, improves insulin sensitivity, increases satiety, and reduces fat storage. Foods containing resistant starch include beans, potatoes, slightly green bananas, split peas, barley, and brown rice.

Dietary fibers, or long chains of complex carbohydrates, include the parts of the plant that are indigestible. Fibers can be categorized into soluble and insoluble.

Soluble fiber can be dissolved in water, forming a gel-like substance and is found in oats, barley, beans, peas, apples, citrus fruits, carrots, and seaweed. Consuming soluble fiber lowers serum cholesterol levels and improves blood glucose control.

Insoluble fiber improves digestion and bowel health, increases satiety, and helps pull out toxins from the body. Foods high in insoluble fiber include fibrous vegetables like asparagus and celery, wheat bran, whole grains, and nuts.

DEFINITION

Soluble fiber is the water-soluble form of dietary fiber that has an affinity for water, either dissolving or swelling to form a gel. **Insoluble fiber** is not soluble in water and consists mainly of lignin, cellulose, and hemicelluloses.

The health benefits of dietary fiber go far beyond digestive health. Eating adequate amounts of soluble and insoluble fiber (present only in plant foods) helps control rates of digestion and sugar absorption, removes heavy metals like mercury and excess sex hormones, enhances weight loss, and prevents colorectal cancer. (See Chapter 4 for more details.)

Refined Versus Whole Carbs

Now, here's the center of all the carb confusion. Comparing refined and whole carbohydrates is critical when talking about eating for health. According to the U.S. Food and Drug Administration (FDA), a *whole grain* is a cereal grain consisting of the "intact, ground, cracked, or flaked fruit whose principal components—the starchy endosperm, germ, and bran—are present in the same relative proportions as they exist in the intact grain."

DEFINITION

Whole grains are derived from the seeds of grasses and include rice, oats, rye, wheat, wild rice, quinoa, barley, buckwheat, bulgur, corn, millet, amaranth, and sorghum.

Whole grains are filled with healthy complex carbs, fiber, protein, vitamins, and minerals. They have zero cholesterol and are low in fat. They meet all our nutritional needs except vitamins A, C, B_{12}, and D and are considered essential in a health-promoting diet. They've been shown to decrease cholesterol and blood sugar levels, as well as lower risk of chronic diseases such as colon cancer, heart disease, and type 2 diabetes. Societies have survived and thrived on a whole-grain–based diet since the beginning of recorded history.

Refined grains, on the other hand, are the end result of processing whole grains. The bran and germ have been removed, leaving only the endosperm. These end products are stripped of vitamins, minerals, and fiber. A diet high in refined products leads to increased risk of chronic disease and supports the confusing misinterpretation of the benefits of a high-carb diet. In other words, a diet high in *refined* carbs does indeed lead to weight gain and illness (as the rumors suggest). However, a diet based on *whole* grains improves health and optimizes weight control. Thus, it's not carbs after all. Instead, it's the source of carbs that matters most.

MIXED GREENS

Dr. John McDougall teaches that humans are starch-eaters and explains how all large populations of trim, healthy people throughout written human history have obtained the bulk of their calories from starch. He also offers current examples of thriving starch-eaters, including Japanese and Chinese in Asia eating sweet potatoes, buckwheat, and rice; Incas in South America eating potatoes; Mayans and Aztecs in Central America eating corn; and Egyptians in the Middle East eating wheat. For more information, see Appendix D.

The Glycemic Index and Glycemic Load

You've probably noticed a lot of talk lately about the glycemic index. But how important is this carbohydrate measuring system? And is it true or just hype?

Developed to help diabetics improve blood sugar control, the glycemic index is a measurement from 0 to 100 that ranks carbs based on how quickly they're converted into blood sugar (glycemia) after they're consumed. Typically, the dose of carbs used to determine the glycemic index is 50 grams, which is then compared to the glycemic response to 50 grams of pure glucose. Foods above 70 are considered high glycemic. These include white bread, watermelon, baked potato, and popcorn. Foods lower than 55, including potato chips, peanuts, honey, and pizza, are categorized as low on the glycemic scale. The lower the number, the less impact the food has on the blood glucose spike. Although blood glucose stability is important for the general population to watch, it's of particular concern for diabetics, who must monitor their blood glucose levels carefully.

Using the glycemic index as an effective tool is controversial for several reasons. Depending on the stage at which a food is ripened or how it's prepared, a wide variation in values is possible. Also, measurements are performed on single items, and the overall result changes when that item is eaten with other foods. Furthermore, glycemic response to foods is subject to individual differences.

An improved version of the glycemic index is the *glycemic load*. A more functional and specific scale, the glycemic load takes the glycemic index an extra step to consider actual intake. It's not practical to assume you'll eat 50 grams of a food each time—unless you typically sit down to 4 slices of bread, $1\frac{1}{2}$ pounds of carrots, $2\frac{1}{2}$ small bananas, or $4\frac{1}{2}$ cups of strawberries. To calculate the glycemic load of a food or a meal, multiply the glycemic index by the carbohydrate content per serving and then divide by 100.

Although some studies suggest a low glycemic load diet may help with weight loss, blood sugar control, and chronic disease prevention, other factors also play a role. Body weight, quality of food consumed, and frequency of exercise also contribute.

Ultimately, a whole-food, plant-based diet optimizes blood sugar control, so you don't need to be overly concerned with measurement tools such as the glycemic index and glycemic load. Just enjoy whole-plant foods, and you'll never have to count, measure, or weigh again!

Powerful Protein

Protein is considered the superhero of macronutrients because of its crucial role in most—if not all—structural and functional mechanisms of the human body. This powerhouse constitutes a part of every cell in the body—muscle, organs, hair, nails, skin, teeth, ligaments, cartilage, and tendons. It's also a component of enzymes, membranes, antibodies, hemoglobin, and some hormones. Protein does everything from compose muscle tissue to fight illness. Although it's not as efficient as carbohydrates, protein is also a source of energy.

MIXED GREENS

In 1839, Gerrit Jan Mulder named the first nutrient "protein," from the Greek word *proteios,* meaning "strength of mind and body." He also commented, "It is highly admirable that the principal substance of all animals is immediately drawn from the plants. It signifies an economy of nature in her means that is wonderful and sublime."

However, just because protein is vital to our health and development doesn't mean more is better. We seem to be obsessed with consuming enough these days, even though research shows we require only about 10 percent of our daily total calories to come from protein.

All About Amino Acids

Amino acids are the building blocks of protein. What distinguishes protein from carbs and fat is the inclusion of nitrogen to the carbon, hydrogen, and oxygen atoms in its makeup. From a total of 20 amino acids, protein is assembled from strings of amino acids in different sequences. Your body is unable to manufacture nine of these amino acids, known as essential amino acids, so you must get them from your diet. Your body can produce the other 11 amino acids.

Under most circumstances, your body is able to synthesize the "conditionally essential" amino acids. Sometimes, though, metabolic demands are higher and your body can't make enough. That's when it becomes necessary for you to get these amino acids from your diet.

The following list breaks down all 20 amino acids into their respective categories based on whether or not they're required in your diet. The essential amino acids must be consumed to create the nonessential amino acids.

Essential:

Histidine	Phenylalanine
Isoleucine	Threonine
Leucine	Tryptophan
Lysine	Valine
Methionine	

Conditionally essential:

Arginine	Glycine
Cysteine	Proline
Glutamine	Tyrosine

Nonessential:

Alanine   Glutamic acid

Asparagine   Serine

Aspartic acid

When you consume protein, your body breaks it down into individual amino acids and stores them in a pool. When a protein needs to be built, the body restrings the amino acids together in the order required to make whatever protein is necessary at the time. It's quite a clever and efficient system!

Debunking Protein Myths

Often, the first question herbivores hear when someone discovers their diet is, "Where do you get your protein?" My favorite response is, "The same place gorillas, elephants, water buffalo, and horses get theirs!"

Somehow people assume that protein comes from only animal products and that anyone avoiding them will be deficient. That's a myth! Not only does the plant world provide abundant protein sources, but we don't need to eat vast quantities of the nutrient to maintain superior health. Consider the fact that the very first food created specifically to nourish an infant during the stage in life when humans grow the most and at the fastest rate is low in protein. Human breast milk contains only 5 percent of its total calories from protein.

According to the Institute of Medicine's Food and Nutrition Board, the Acceptable Macronutrient Distribution Range (AMDR) for protein is 10 to 35 percent of total calories. However, if you look at the data from *The China Study* and the World Health Organization's Food and Agricultural Organization, we actually need only 5 or 6 percent of our total calories from protein to replace what we lose every day.

To take that a step further, plenty of research shows that once protein intake increases to levels above 10 percent—specifically from animal sources—disease processes begin. This suggests it's best to maintain protein consumption at approximately 10 percent of total calories.

If you're eating enough calories from whole foods, having a diet too low in protein is impossible. Virtually all whole-plant foods include protein. For example, bananas contain 5 percent of their total calories from protein, white potatoes have 8 percent, and brown rice has 9 percent. These foods are categorized as carbs, yet they meet the requirements to replace necessary protein.

Furthermore, some plant foods are very high in protein, including beans, legumes, nuts, and seeds. Lentils have 36 percent, and, believe it or not, leafy green vegetables have almost half their total calories from protein! The only way to become deficient in protein is either not to eat enough calories or to eat primarily processed and refined foods. Ultimately, if you stick to eating whole-plant foods, you don't need to worry about getting enough protein.

Protein combining is another myth. It's based on the notion that the body requires all nine essential amino acids present in every meal. Animal proteins have a reputation for being complete proteins because they contain all the essential amino acids. Plant proteins don't. However, even though they may not appear together in the same food item, every single amino acid is represented in the plant kingdom. Additionally, our body requires and utilizes amino acids—not intact proteins.

DEFINITION

Protein combining was a theory that began in the 1970s that nutrition experts taught to ensure adequate amounts of all the essential amino acids were consumed. Certain foods were recommended to be eaten together at the same meal (grains and legumes, for example) to prevent protein deficiency. This antiquated method is no longer promoted because it's been confirmed that your body can make proteins out of pooled amino acids as long as you eat a variety of plant foods and meet your energy needs.

This idea for combining foods was instigated by Frances Moore Lappé's 1971 book *Diet for a Small Planet*. The concept has since been repudiated by medical experts, including the author herself. Ultimately, the human body is much more intelligent than we give it credit for. It's able to pool together all the amino acids it absorbs from food and re-create the proteins it requires as necessary.

How Much Do We Really Require?

The Recommended Daily Allowance (RDA) for protein set by the U.S. Department of Agriculture is 0.8 gram per kilogram of bodyweight per day (g/kg/day) for adults 19 years old and above. The RDAs for children are higher on a gram-per-bodyweight basis than for adults:

Ages 1 to 3 years	1.05 g/kg/day
Ages 4 to 13 years	0.95 g/kg/day
Ages 14 to 18 years	0.85 g/kg/day

RDAs for protein also are increased for pregnant and lactating women:

| Pregnant | 1.1 g/kg/day |
| Lactating | 1.3 g/kg/day |

HEALTHY HINT

To figure out how many kilograms you weigh, simply divide your weight in pounds by 2.2. For example, a 130-pound female weighs 59 kilograms (130 ÷ 2.2 = 59).

But wait! Here's some fabulous news: following a whole-food, plant-based diet automatically gives you perfect amounts of protein, carbs, and fat. As long as you consume a variety of foods, you don't need to worry about calculating, weighing, measuring, or counting. This is one of the many benefits associated with eating a healthy veg diet. So put down your calculator and breathe a sigh of relief. Eat a variety of whole-plant foods, and you'll be naturally macronutrient balanced!

Super Sources of Protein

Sources of protein are abundant in the plant kingdom. Ample quantities and varieties of amino acids come packaged with phytochemicals, antioxidants, fiber, vitamins, and minerals. In animal flesh, eggs, and dairy products, protein comes along with saturated fat, cholesterol, and none of the above-mentioned health-promoting nutrients. The following table shares some terrific plant-based sources of protein.

PLANT PITFALL

Including excessive amounts of protein not only is unnecessary, but it also can be dangerous. The kidneys, which metabolize protein, have to work hard to break down the nitrogenous waste that accrues with a high protein intake. Overworking the kidneys with large quantities of protein can lead to kidney stones and other, more serious diseases.

Excellent Plant Protein Sources

Food	% Calories from Protein	Protein per Serving
Banana, 1 medium	4.6	1.2g
Brown rice, 1 cup cooked	8.5	4.9g
Barley, pearled, 1 cup cooked	9.4	16.4g
Quinoa, ½ cup cooked	14.0	11.1g
Whole-wheat bread, 1 slice	15.7	2.4g
Chickpeas, 1 cup cooked	21.6	14.5g
Lentils, 1 cup cooked	31.0	17.9g
Soy milk, 1 cup	33.4	6.6g
Broccoli, raw, ½ cup	43.3	1.3g
Tofu, raw, firm, ½ cup	43.5	19.9g
Spinach, frozen, ½ cup	44.4	3.0g

Fat: Fact and Fiction

Low fat, high fat, trans fat, saturated fat—sometimes it's difficult to keep straight all the kinds of fat, let alone know whether they're good or bad for you!

Let's make this simple so that fat makes sense. You do need to eat some fat every day. Because some fats are healthful and others are harmful, I can help you distinguish the two. It's easy to eat adequate amounts of healthy fat from whole-plant foods—and, as a bonus, it's difficult to find unhealthy fats in these foods! Here's yet another reason to celebrate the beauty of the whole-food, plant-based diet!

The Facts About Fats

Your body requires dietary fats, also known as lipids, to perform several functions. First, fat helps with the absorption of fat-soluble vitamins, minerals, and phytochemicals like carotenoids. Fat is also a major source of energy, like carbohydrates and protein. However, at 9 calories per gram (kcal/g), fat offers more than twice the amount of energy because both carbs and protein supply just 4 kcal/g.

Fat also provides essential fatty acids (linoleic acid and alpha-linolenic acid) that the body can't produce on its own and that must be consumed via diet. A fatty acid is to fat what a saccharide is to sugar and amino acid to protein. These single components bind to a glycerol backbone to be transported and stored throughout the body as triglycerides. They're classified based on the length of the fatty acid chains and on their chemical composition. Additionally, some fatty acids act as precursors that help with coagulation (blood clotting), inflammation, and gene expression.

Dietary fat is found in both plant and animal sources. The degree of saturation determines its physical state. The more saturated the fatty acid, the more solid it appears at room temperature. Plant fats tend to have lower melting points than do animal fats and are liquid at room temperature—think oils. The exceptions to this rule in the plant kingdom are the tropical oils: coconut, palm kernel, and palm. These oils are high in saturated fatty acids, and therefore are solid at room temperature. Also, trans fatty acids are chemically altered in the lab to be solid at room temperature.

The USDA has not set an RDA, adequate intake (AI), or upper limit (UL) for total fat intake (except for infants). Instead, it uses the AMDR of 20 to 35 percent for adults. Research confirms that eating a diet high in fat promotes excess weight, obesity, and chronic disease. It's associated with higher blood cholesterol levels, breast and bowel cancer rates, and heart disease.

However, evidence is beginning to show that the *amount* of fat consumed is not as important as the *source* of that fat. Fats derived from whole-plant foods are either neutral or health-protective; fats from animal products and processed vegetable oils are more strongly associated with chronic disease.

Types of Fats

Here are the types of fats found in food:

Monounsaturated fatty acids (MUFA) are fatty acids that have one (mono) double bond in its structure. They are liquid at room temperature but may become cloudy and thickened in the refrigerator. Found in olives, peanuts, avocados, pecans, almonds, their oils, and canola oil, MUFAs are heart healthy.

Polyunsaturated fatty acids (PUFA) contain at least two double bonds and are usually liquid both at room temperature and in the refrigerator. PUFAs make up both the omega-3 (alpha-linolenic acid, ALA) and omega-6 (linoleic acid, LA) essential fatty acids. These are required for growth, reproduction, skin function, cholesterol metabolism, and cellular communication. Found in walnuts, flaxseeds, hempseeds, vegetable oils (especially canola, soybean, and flaxseed), fish, and marine oils, PUFAs protect against coronary heart disease, certain cancers, and other inflammatory diseases.

Saturated fatty acids (SFA) have no double bonds and are primarily found in animal products. Tropical oils are the only plant sources with SFAs. SFAs are known to raise blood cholesterol and promote heart disease. Consuming SFAs is unnecessary, and, in fact, the Food and Nutrition Board of the Institute of Medicine recommends eating "as little as possible while consuming a nutritionally adequate diet."

Trans fatty acids (TFA) are a relatively new invention. These unsaturated fats are created in a lab by a process called hydrogenation and are possibly the most harmful type of fat we can consume. They are used to solidify a product and increase the shelf life of processed, fried, and fast foods. In the meantime, TFAs minimize the shelf life of your health! If you see the words *hydrogenated* or *partially hydrogenated* on an ingredient list, put down the product and quickly walk away!

Triglycerides (TG) are the chemical form taken by most fats both in the body and in food. When not used immediately, any excess calories consumed in a meal are transformed into TGs for transport and storage in fat cells.

The Cholesterol Conundrum

Cholesterol is a waxy substance that naturally occurs in all parts of the body and is required for normal function. It's found in cell walls or membranes throughout the entire body and is necessary to produce many hormones, vitamin D, and the bile acids that help to digest fat.

Only a small amount of cholesterol is essential for all the roles it plays in the body, and the liver produces all your body really needs. Your liver makes about 800 to 1,000 milligrams per day, so it's not necessary to consume any other cholesterol from your diet!

Excessive amounts of cholesterol in the bloodstream lead to atherosclerosis, a condition in which fat and cholesterol are deposited in the walls of the arteries throughout the body. This process eventually generates the signs and symptoms of cardiovascular disease. Because cholesterol is made exclusively in the liver, it's found only in animal products.

HEALTHY HINT

Phytosterols, or plant sterols found in small amounts in all whole-plant foods, are compounds similar in structure to cholesterol. But they have been shown to help block the absorption of cholesterol in the gut.

The Good, the Bad, and the Ugly

Let's start with the good fats: MUFAs and PUFAs. MUFAs have no negative effects and even slightly beneficial effects on health. Evidence suggests MUFAs might reduce blood pressure, enhance blood flow, and minimally affect blood cholesterol, making them heart healthy. PUFAs are also beneficial overall, especially when they replace TFAs and SFAs in the diet. Certain PUFAs (the essential fatty acids) are required for human survival.

SFAs and TFAs, on the other hand, are the bad and the ugly of the fat world. The bad increases the risk of chronic diseases, including coronary artery disease, some types of cancers, kidney disease, type 2 diabetes, and gallstones. Two to four times more damaging than SFAs, the ugly win the gold medal for the unhealthiest fat. Harmful and disease-promoting, TFAs increase heart disease risk, interfere with liver function, increase the potential of having low-birth-weight babies, interrupt essential fatty acid metabolism, and worsen insulin resistance. TFAs are found primarily in processed and deep-fried fast foods.

So what does all this mean? Avoid animal products and processed and deep-fried foods. Instead, consume a variety of whole-plant foods, and you'll minimize your risk of developing chronic disease.

Ideal Intake

Debate rages among leading experts in plant-based nutrition about exactly how much total dietary fat intake is ideal. Data indicate that a low-fat diet, with 10 percent of total calories from fat, is optimal for reversing heart disease and other chronic diseases.

Other research confirms that eating a diet with a higher percentage of fat—15 to 25 percent and even greater than 40 percent of total calories—is healthful as long as the sources for that fat are whole foods (avocados, olives, nuts, and seeds). In fact, no research currently shows these fats to be harmful while consumed on a whole-food, plant-based diet. The same can't be said for a high intake of oils and animal fat, which has been shown to cause chronic disease.

Everyone is unique, and bodies respond differently depending on genetics, health status, exercise, stress, and other factors. So how do you decide what the ideal intake is for you? First, be certain you're getting all your fat from whole-food sources. And choose the amount of fat that will enable you to maintain a whole-food, plant-based diet throughout your life. It's as simple as that.

Essential Fatty Acid Balancing Act

The biochemistry of essential fatty acid metabolism is extremely complex. Essentially, the Standard American Diet (SAD) supplies excessive amounts of omega-6 fatty acids and inadequate amounts of omega-3 fatty acids. Omega-3 fatty acids help prevent disease, and overconsumption of omega-6 fatty acids promotes inflammation (a disease-supporting process). Thus, balancing the two is an art worth mastering! Although deficiency is rare, much research suggests protective effects of maintaining fatty acid harmony. Following are the fundamentals you need to know to become a pro.

Foods provide two essential fatty acids: linoleic acid (LA, an omega-6 fatty acid) and alpha-linolenic acid (ALA, an omega-3 fatty acid). Your body can convert these into other compounds needed to perform various functions. LA is ubiquitous in the food world. Not consuming enough would be challenging. In fact, most people are consuming way too much. LA easily converts into highly unsaturated fatty acids (HUFAs), which are vastly active in the body and have powerful health benefits.

In contrast, ALA has a hard time converting into its final products—eicosapentaenoic acid (EPA) and docosahexaenoic acid (DHA), two extremely important long-chain fatty acids. You need an adequate supply of EPA and DHA to meet your essential fat requirements. However, plant-based eaters have no direct source for EPA and DHA in their diet. EPA and DHA come from animal products only, namely, fish, fish oils, and specialty dairy and egg products. We have to rely on the conversion from ALA to meet our goals. So what's an herbivore to do?

PLANT PITFALL

Fish oil is a commonly used supplement for people trying to consume adequate omega-3 fatty acids. Although rich in EPA and DHA, it also happens to be a highly concentrated source of contaminants. Fish contain large doses of heavy metals (lead, mercury, and cadmium) and industrial pollutants (PCBs, DDT, and dioxin)—all of which are carcinogenic, or cancer-promoting.

Well, several variables impact the conversion of ALA to EPA and DHA. First, you need to consume the recommended Adequate Intake levels of ALA—1.6 grams for men and 1.1 grams for women.

Another important factor is to maintain the ratio of omega-6 and omega-3 fatty acids between 2:1 and 4:1. In other words, you should consume twice to four times the amount of omega-6 fatty acids than omega-3 fatty acids. For comparison, herbivores typically consume a ratio of 14:1 to 20:1, which is a far cry from a healthy proportion!

Whole foods high in omega-6 fatty acids include sesame seeds, tahini, sunflower seeds, pumpkin seeds, soybeans (a.k.a. edamame), wheat germ, and tofu. Good sources for omega-3 fatty acids are flaxseeds, hempseeds, leafy green vegetables, walnuts, and seaweed. In fact, you can get a daily allotment of ALA from just a tablespoon of ground flaxseed! Foods with a healthy balance of omega-6 to omega-3 fatty acids include flaxseeds, leafy green vegetables, hempseeds, and walnuts.

The following table provides specific amounts of whole-plant foods you can eat to reach your daily Adequate Intake of ALA omega-3 fatty acids, whether you're a man or a woman.

Meeting Your ALA Needs

Food	ALA Content	Amount Needed to Provide 1.6g ALA	Amount Needed to Provide 1.1g ALA
Grapeseed oil, 1 TB.	0.014g	114 TB.	79 TB.
Olive oil, 1 TB.	0.103g	15.5 TB.	10.7 TB.
Avocado oil, 1 TB.	0.134g	12 TB.	8 TB.
Kale, 1 cup cooked	0.134g	11.9 cups	8.2 cups
Collards, 1 cup cooked	0.177g	9 cups	6.2 cups
Tempeh, $\frac{1}{2}$ cup	0.183g	4.4 cups	3 cups
Broccoli, 1 cup cooked	0.186g	8.6 cups	5.9 cups
Tofu, firm, $\frac{1}{2}$ cup	0.228g	3.5 cups	2.4 cups
Black walnuts, 2 TB.	0.312g	0.6 cup	0.4 cup
Soybeans, 1 cup	1.029g	1.6 cups	1.1 cups
Canola oil, 1 TB.	1.279g	1.25 TB.	0.9 TB.
English walnuts, 2 TB.	1.352g	2.4 TB.	1.6 TB.
Walnut oil, 1 TB.	1.414g	1.1 TB.	0.8 TB.
Hempseed oil, 1 TB.	2.240g	0.7 TB.	0.5 TB.
Flaxseeds, ground, 2 TB.	3.194g	1 TB.	0.7 TB.
Flaxseeds, whole*, 2 TB.	3.194g	1 TB.	0.5 TB.
Flaxseed oil, 1 TB.	7.249g	0.2 TB.	0.15 TB.

Flaxseeds cannot be digested whole. Grind before eating.

Further, consume a nutritionally adequate diet by following the guidelines in this book. Diets including TFAs, high amounts of omega-6 fatty acids, and/or alcohol hinder conversion to EPA and DHA.

Finally, for those of you who are pregnant, nursing, highly active, or have diabetes or a metabolic disorder that limits the ability to produce the conversion enzymes, consider taking a direct source of DHA. Vegan microalgae formulas are available to help boost intake. Look for a veg cap version, and take the recommended 100 to 300 milligrams per day.

Whether you're a recovering carbophobe or protein prowler, you can see how ideas have been hyped up and cause mass confusion. Essentially, all food contains some combination of carbs, protein, and fat. Your red flag should go on alert when one of these essential groups of nutrients becomes the focus of attention. You need a lot of whole carbs and some protein and fat to perform your daily functions. When you eat whole-plant foods, you automatically and effortlessly strike the perfect balance.

The Least You Need to Know

- The three macronutrients—carbohydrates, protein, and fat—make up all the calories in your diet and serve uniquely important functions in energy, metabolism, and health.
- Carbohydrates supply the body with the most efficient form of energy and the only source of fuel for the brain. Whole-food sources rich in carbohydrates include the most nutrient-dense foods on the planet: vegetables, fruits, whole grains, and legumes.
- Protein is needed in a smaller amount than commonly thought, and it's impossible to be protein deficient on a whole-food, plant-based diet.
- All amino acids are present in plants and are packaged healthfully alongside fiber, vitamins, minerals, and phytochemicals.
- Fats from whole-food sources provide optimal types and quantities of essential fatty acids, as long as oil and animal fats are eliminated.

Getting Your Vitamins and Minerals

In This Chapter

- Everything you need to know about vitamins and minerals
- Fat-soluble versus water-soluble vitamins
- The big, the tiny, and the necessary minerals

Now that you're familiar with the macronutrients in Chapter 2, it's time to introduce you to the little guys. Micronutrients are a group of essential substances required in small quantities for normal metabolism. Even though you need only a trivial amount of these nutrients, they're an extremely critical component of your day-to-day functioning.

Versatile Vitamins

Thirteen vitamins quietly hide in the foods you consume, awaiting absorption in the GI tract so they can kick into gear and perform their jobs. Vitamins are divided into two categories: water-soluble and fat-soluble. They are separated based on their physical properties and how they act inside the body. Of the 13, 4 are fat-soluble vitamins, while the remaining 9 are water-soluble.

MIXED GREENS

The Food and Nutrition Board of the National Academy of Science's Institute of Medicine sets the Recommended Dietary Allowances (RDA). These guidelines suggest the dietary intake level sufficient to meet the nutrient requirements of nearly all (97 to 98 percent) healthy individuals in a particular life stage and gender group. After an explosion of nutrition discoveries, an additional group of guidelines was established in 1998 called the Dietary Reference Intakes (DRIs). DRIs include RDAs as the target intake; adequate intake (AI); tolerable upper limit (UL) of certain nutrients; and estimated average requirement (EAR). All these recommendations are based on the objective of "minimizing risk for chronic disease."

Fat- Versus Water-Soluble Vitamins

Fat-soluble vitamins, which include A, D, E, and K, require fat for absorption, hence the name. They're stored in your body's tissues and are excreted via the feces. Excess doses can lead to toxicity, and deficiency is possible if inadequate fat is consumed or absorbed.

Water-soluble vitamins, on the other hand, consist of the eight B-complex vitamins and vitamin C. They can be dissolved in water, are not stored in the body, and are eliminated in the urine. Therefore, you need to replenish them every day. Similarly, they're easily destroyed and washed out during storage, preparation, and cooking, so they need to be cared for delicately.

To reduce their destruction, avoid overcooking foods high in water-soluble vitamins, and steam these foods instead of boiling them. Also be sure to consume raw sources regularly. Keep your produce refrigerated, too. The moment a fruit or vegetable is exposed to oxygen, the vitamins begin to degrade, so use freshly picked produce as often as possible. (Purchase your produce from a farmers' market or community-supported agriculture, or grow a garden of your own—and consume it as quickly as possible!)

Let's take a look at each of the vitamins in a little more detail, starting with the fat-soluble vitamins.

Vitamin A

Vitamin A refers to a group of compounds essential for growth, vision, reproduction, and immune function. Preformed vitamin A is found only in animals, but provitamin carotenoids, found abundantly in fruits and vegetables, can be converted into vitamin A. Even though at least 600 of them exist in nature, only about 50 can be converted into retinol, the active form of vitamin A. Beta-carotene is the most active and most commonly known of these carotenoids. Carotenoids come in a spectrum of reds, oranges, and yellows in pigment; however, they can be found hidden by the dark-green chlorophyll color in leafy green vegetables.

Carotenoids are powerful antioxidants. Lycopene, one of the most potent antioxidants in the carotenoid family, is known to prevent and treat prostate cancer. It's also effective against other cancers, heart disease, and age-related macular degeneration. Cook your lycopene sources (found abundantly in tomatoes) to enhance its availability.

Similarly, high doses of lutein and zeaxanthin—other carotenoids—reduce the risk of age-related macular degeneration and cataracts. These carotenoids, also found in leafy green vegetables, require fat for absorption. If you're following a low-fat diet or have any issues with absorption, you may be at risk for deficiency of these important nutrients. I suggest eating your leafy greens and tomatoes with a bit of fat, like nuts, seeds, or avocados.

Beta-carotene, one of the most well-known carotenoids, is found in foods with orange and yellow hues. This carotenoid works synergistically with vitamin E to support health protection. High doses can lead to a yellowing of the skin, a harmless condition. However, when taken in high doses via supplements, beta-carotene increases the risk of cancer and heart disease in people who smoke or drink alcohol excessively.

Not surprisingly, carotenoid intake tends to be high in herbivores. The RDA for vitamin A is 900 micrograms for men and 700 micrograms for women. Pregnant women need 770 micrograms a day and 1,300 micrograms when lactating. Excellent plant-based sources of provitamin A include tomato, pumpkin, sweet potato, butternut squash, kale, spinach, cantaloupe, mango, and apricots.

The following table gives you the vitamin A content found in certain foods.

Vitamin A

Food	Vitamin A (mcg RAE)
Tomato juice, $\frac{1}{2}$ cup	28
Nectarine, 1 medium	50
Milk, whole, $\frac{1}{2}$ cup	56
Broccoli, $\frac{1}{2}$ cup	60
Cow's milk, 2%, $\frac{1}{2}$ cup	67
Cheddar cheese, 1 oz.	75

continues

Vitamin A *continued*

Food	Vitamin A (mcg RAE)
Tomato, 1 medium	76
Mango, 1 medium	80
Apricots, raw, 3	101
Cantaloupe, $\frac{1}{2}$ cup	135
Collard greens, $\frac{1}{2}$ cup	148
Papaya, 1 medium	167
Bok choy, $\frac{1}{2}$ cup	180
Mustard greens, $\frac{1}{2}$ cup	221
Swiss chard, $\frac{1}{2}$ cup	268
Beet greens, $\frac{1}{2}$ cup	276
Dandelion greens, $\frac{1}{2}$ cup	356
Spinach, $\frac{1}{2}$ cup	472
Butternut squash, $\frac{1}{2}$ cup	572
Carrots, $\frac{1}{2}$ cup	665
Pumpkin, canned, $\frac{1}{2}$ cup	953
Sweet potatoes, $\frac{1}{2}$ cup	1,291
Kale, $\frac{1}{2}$ cup	2,443

Vitamin D

Vitamin D has become the vitamin du jour as studies focus on an almost universal insufficiency. Currently, 70 to 97 percent of the U.S. population is lacking in vitamin D! This shouldn't be taken lightly. Every cell in the body contains vitamin D receptors, indicating its importance for optimal overall functioning. Two commonly known functions of vitamin D include maintaining blood levels of calcium and phosphorus and supporting the cardiovascular system. Your blood level of 25-hydroxyvitamin D (the appropriate test to request from your doctor) should be at least 35 ng/mL; optimum levels are 50 ng/mL and above.

Normally, skin produces vitamin D when exposed to sunlight. A cholesterol compound in your skin called 7-dehydrocholesterol is activated by UVB sun ray exposure. After a visit to the liver and then the kidneys, this compound is transformed into 1, 25-dihydroxyvitamin D, the biologically active form of vitamin D. At this point, vitamin D is acting as a true hormone that gets busy on many fronts performing structural and functional jobs throughout the body.

People who live farther away from the equator have an increased incidence of vitamin D deficiency and are, therefore, at an amplified risk for many chronic diseases. Preformed vitamin D is found only in animal products, specifically in fatty fish and their liver oils, milk, beef liver, and egg yolks. Because vitamin D is hard to come by nutritionally, foods like dairy and plant milks, fruit juices, cereals, breads, nutrition bars, and pastas are fortified with vitamin D.

Herbivores and carnivores are at the same risk for vitamin D deficiency, so it's important for everyone to get their vitamin D levels checked by a blood test. The results can help you determine whether you need to consider properly increasing your sun exposure and/or adding a supplement. Populations with darker skin, breastfed infants, people with limited sun exposure, obese individuals, elderly people, and anyone with gastrointestinal absorption issues are at higher risk for vitamin D deficiency. Low vitamin D levels are consistently associated with most chronic diseases, including many cancers, heart disease, osteoporosis, type 2 diabetes, and autoimmune diseases.

How much vitamin D should you consume daily? The RDA is 600 IU per day for all adult populations from a year to 70 years of age. After 71, the RDA increases to 800 IU. Many leading researchers believe higher doses are necessary to sustain optimal levels of vitamin D. (See Chapter 10 to learn more about how to ensure adequate blood vitamin D levels.)

The following table gives you the vitamin D content found in certain foods.

Vitamin D

Food	Vitamin D (mcg)
Fortified margarine, 1 tsp.	0.5
Eggs, 1 large	0.6
Fortified plant milk, 1 cup	2.5 to 3.0
Fortified cow's milk, 2%, 1 cup	2.9

> **MIXED GREENS**
>
> Is vitamin D a vitamin or a hormone? It's both! Because it's obtained from the diet and required for survival, vitamin D is like a vitamin. By definition, however, a vitamin can't be created by the body. A hormone, on the other hand, is a chemical substance formed in one organ and carried via the blood to another organ, where it exerts functional effects. When the sun's ultraviolet B (UVB) rays hit the skin, they kick off a chain reaction that ultimately generates the active form of vitamin D. That reaction implies that vitamin D is also a hormone. But because it's found naturally in foods, the name "vitamin D" is the accepted term for this important hormone.

Vitamin E

Vitamin E exists in eight different forms, but only alpha-tocopherol is active and can meet human requirements. This form of vitamin E is a potent antioxidant. With deficiency—which is rare, thanks to its presence in many foods—red blood cells become fragile and increased free radical damage occurs, leaving the body susceptible to damage due to oxidation. Although you need oxygen to stay alive, oxygen can cause an imbalance in your cells, where reactive compounds (free radicals) outweigh the presence of antioxidants. High exposure to free radicals and oxidation initiates many disease processes, like heart disease and cancer, and speeds up aging. (See Chapter 4 for more details on this process.) Antioxidants, like vitamin E and the carotenoids, halt oxidation.

In addition to its antioxidant activities, vitamin E also participates in immune function, regulating gene expression and other metabolic processes. With ample amounts, vitamin E helps keep the inner (endothelial) lining of the blood vessels smooth. This keeps blood cell components from sticking to it, which helps prevent plaque build-up. Another heart-helpful task vitamin E performs is boosting two enzymes that increase the release of a compound called prostacyclin. Prostacyclin prevents blood clots and keeps the blood vessels open and flowing.

The RDA for vitamin E is 15 milligrams per day for both adult men and women. For children age 1 to 3 years, 3 milligrams is recommended, and from age 4 to 8, the RDA increases to 7 milligrams. Children age 9 to 13 years require 11 milligrams. With lactation, vitamin E RDA increases to 19 milligrams per day. Plant sources of vitamin E include avocados, wheat germ, sunflower seeds, almonds and almond butter, peanuts and peanut butter, pumpkin, soybeans, olives, and leafy green vegetables.

The following table gives you the vitamin E content found in certain foods.

Vitamin E

Food	Vitamin E (mg ATE)
Pear, 1 medium	0.28
Soybeans, $\frac{1}{2}$ cup	0.3
Apple, 1 medium	0.33
Kohlrabi, $\frac{1}{2}$ cup cooked	0.43
Quinoa, $\frac{1}{2}$ cup	0.58
Olive oil, 1 tsp.	0.65
Peanut oil, 1 tsp.	0.71
Canola oil, 1 tsp.	0.79
Mustard greens, $\frac{1}{2}$ cup cooked	0.85
Kelp, $\frac{1}{2}$ cup cooked	0.9
Pumpkin, canned, $\frac{1}{2}$ cup cooked	1.3
Turnip greens, $\frac{1}{2}$ cup cooked	1.35
Swiss chard, $\frac{1}{2}$ cup cooked	1.6
Pomegranate, 1 medium	1.7
Sunflower oil, 1 tsp.	1.85
Spinach, $\frac{1}{2}$ cup cooked	1.9
Avocado, raw, $\frac{1}{2}$	2
Mango, 1 medium	2.3
Wheat germ, 2 TB.	2.5
Peanut butter, 2 TB.	2.9
Peanuts, $\frac{1}{4}$ cup	3
Hazelnuts, $\frac{1}{4}$ cup	4.32
Wheat germ oil, 1 tsp.	6.72
Almonds, $\frac{1}{4}$ cup	7.8
Almond butter, 2 TB.	8.3

Vitamin K

Vitamin K plays an essential role in blood clotting. In fact, its name originates from the German word *koagulation*, which is what vitamin K helps regulate in the blood. When you get a wound, vitamin K helps the blood clot and begin the healing process. On the flip side, you don't want to produce unnecessary, potentially fatal clots in your bloodstream because they lead to obstructive heart attacks, peripheral vascular disease, and strokes. Vitamin K regulates coagulation to keep you clotting only when necessary.

With the drug Warfarin (or brand name Coumadin), vitamin K becomes a balancing act. If you're on this drug for anticoagulant purposes, you need to maintain a consistent intake of vitamin K to allow the drug to work properly. Ask your physician to moderate your dosage while allowing you to consume adequate green vegetables to optimize your overall health.

PLANT PITFALL

People who are on anticoagulant drug therapy (which inhibits the clotting action of vitamin K) need to monitor their vitamin K intake carefully.

Vitamin K also assists in bone metabolism, mitigating the breakdown of bone minerals by osteoclasts and strengthening the composition of the bone. Low vitamin K levels in the blood are associated with low bone mineral density and higher rates of fractures.

Although deficiency is rare, it can affect breastfed newborn infants (which is why newborns in the United States are given a vitamin K injection right after birth), as well as adults who are suffering from malabsorption or are chronically taking antibiotics. Normally, the bacteria that live in your gut produce vitamin K. That's why the previously mentioned populations are at risk for inhibiting that process. Deficiency can lead to decreased bone mineral density and bleeding.

Fortunately, vitamin K is omnipresent in the plant kingdom, especially in anything green. There are two forms of vitamin K available. The type known as menaquinone is found in bacteria. The plant version is called phylloquinone, and this is the primary dietary source for vitamin K. Like the other fat-soluble vitamins, foods rich in vitamin K need to be consumed with some fat. So add nuts, seeds, olives, and/or avocado to your green veggies to enhance absorption.

For adults 19 years and older, the daily adequate intake of vitamin K is 120 micrograms for men and 90 micrograms for women. Leafy green vegetables are excellent sources for vitamin K, as are broccoli, asparagus, lentils, and peas.

The following table gives you the vitamin K content found in certain foods.

Vitamin K

Food	Vitamin K (mcg)
Miso paste, 1 TB.	15
Romaine lettuce, raw, $\frac{1}{2}$ cup	24
Asparagus, $\frac{1}{2}$ cup cooked	45
Cabbage, $\frac{1}{2}$ cup cooked	81
Brussels sprouts, $\frac{1}{2}$ cup cooked	109
Broccoli, $\frac{1}{2}$ cup cooked	110
Turnip greens, $\frac{1}{2}$ cup cooked	265
Collard greens, $\frac{1}{2}$ cup cooked	418
Spinach, $\frac{1}{2}$ cup cooked	444
Kale, $\frac{1}{2}$ cup cooked	531

Thiamin (Vitamin B$_1$)

Now let's switch to the water-soluble vitamins, starting with thiamin. Also known as vitamin B$_1$, thiamin acts as a *coenzyme* in the metabolism of carbohydrates and branched-chain amino acids. In other words, it helps convert carbs into energy.

DEFINITION

Coenzymes are small, nonprotein molecules that enhance the action of an enzyme.

Thiamin deficiency is common in alcoholics. Many mechanisms contribute to thiamin deficiency in alcoholics, known as Wernicke-Korsakoff syndrome, including decreased intake, impaired absorption and use, and increased demand. Beriberi, a disease caused by thiamin deficiency that can lead to pain, mental confusion, and paralysis, is extremely rare because many foods are fortified with thiamin.

The RDA for thiamin is set at 1.2 and 1.1 milligrams per day in adult men and women, respectively. During pregnancy and lactation, women require 1.4 milligrams a day. Thiamin is found in whole grains such as quinoa, oats, and barley; beans, peas, and other legumes; nutritional yeast; brewer's yeast; winter squash; and tahini.

Riboflavin (Vitamin B$_2$)

Riboflavin, or vitamin B$_2$, plays a vital role as a coenzyme in energy metabolism. It's also important for growth and red blood cell formation. Although uncommon, deficiency can lead to mouth sores, a swollen tongue, inflamed and reddened skin, and a rare form of anemia.

Riboflavin is sensitive; it can be destroyed by sunlight, and substantial amounts can be lost in cooking water during boiling. So keep your produce refrigerated and use that cooking water again for soup!

The adult RDA for riboflavin is 1.3 milligrams for men and 1.1 milligrams for women. The daily requirement increases to 1.4 milligrams during pregnancy and 1.6 milligrams during lactation. Sources include nutritional yeast, fortified cereals and plant milks, barley, soybeans, mushrooms, spinach, sea vegetables, and beet greens.

> **MIXED GREENS**
>
> You know when you take a multivitamin and your urine is fluorescent yellow? You can thank riboflavin for that!

Niacin (Vitamin B$_3$)

Niacin, or vitamin B$_3$, also contributes to energy by metabolizing glucose and fatty acids. (You can see why all these vitamins are in the same B family!) Used in therapeutic doses (think large), niacin helps raise HDL cholesterol levels. Niacin is also necessary in the production of DNA.

Pellagra is the disease associated with a deficiency of niacin. Symptoms of pellagra include confusion, delusion, diarrhea, inflamed mucous membranes, and scaly skin sores.

RDA for niacin in adults is 16 and 14 milligrams per day for men and women, respectively. An increase to 18 milligrams during pregnancy and then down to 17 milligrams per day for lactation is recommended. Plant-based niacin sources include fortified cereals, nutritional yeast, barley, rice, peanuts and peanut butter, brewer's yeast, tahini, tempeh, mushrooms, avocados, peas, and potatoes.

Vitamin B_6

Vitamin B_6 is comprised of three compounds (pyridoxine, pyridoxal, and pyridoxamine) that are all converted to its active forms, pyridoxal phosphate and pyridoxamine. B_6 functions as a coenzyme for more than 100 different enzymes that are primarily involved in amino acid metabolism. It's also essential for red blood cell metabolism and for keeping blood sugar levels stable. Vitamin B_6 may even have antioxidant properties. This vitamin is required for optimal function of both the nervous and immune systems. Maintaining an adequate consumption of B_6 also protects against heart disease.

Older people and individuals on a poor-quality diet may have suboptimal vitamin B_6 nutritional status. Symptoms of vitamin B_6 deficiency don't appear until later, when intake has been very low for an extended time. Signs of vitamin B_6 deficiency include dermatitis (skin inflammation), glossitis (a sore tongue), depression, confusion, and convulsions.

Adult RDA values vary according to age: from 1.3 milligrams for men and women age 19 to 50, 1.7 milligrams for men over 51, and 1.5 milligrams for women over age 51. During pregnancy, women need 1.9 milligrams daily and 2.0 milligrams daily when lactating. B_6 is found in a wide variety of foods, including fortified cereals, bananas, figs, raisins, chickpeas, lentils, sweet potatoes, tomato juice, avocados, soy products, and brewer's yeast.

The following table gives you the vitamin B_6 content found in certain foods.

Vitamin B_6

Food	Vitamin B_6 (mg)
Asparagus, $1/2$ cup cooked	0.04
Watermelon, $1/2$ cup	0.04
Raisins, $1/2$ cup	0.07
Peas, $1/2$ cup cooked	0.09
Figs, 10	0.09
Nori, dried, 8g	0.1

continues

Vitamin B$_6$ *continued*

Food	Vitamin B$_6$ (mg)
Orange juice, $\frac{1}{2}$ cup	0.1
Sunflower seeds, 2 TB.	0.1
Quinoa, $\frac{1}{2}$ cup cooked	0.11
Chickpeas, $\frac{1}{2}$ cup cooked	0.11
Kidney beans, $\frac{1}{2}$ cup cooked	0.11
Navy beans, $\frac{1}{2}$ cup cooked	0.12
Soy milk, $\frac{1}{2}$ cup	0.12
Winter squash, $\frac{1}{2}$ cup cooked	0.12 to 0.20
Brown rice, $\frac{1}{2}$ cup cooked	0.14
Tomato juice, $\frac{1}{2}$ cup	0.14
Lima beans, $\frac{1}{2}$ cup cooked	0.15
Lentils, $\frac{1}{2}$ cup cooked	0.17
Plantains, $\frac{1}{2}$ cup cooked	0.18
Tempeh, $\frac{1}{2}$ cup cooked	0.18
Pinto beans, $\frac{1}{2}$ cup cooked	0.19
Soybeans, $\frac{1}{2}$ cup cooked	0.20
Spinach, $\frac{1}{2}$ cup cooked	0.22
Potatoes, $\frac{1}{2}$ cup cooked	0.23
Avocado, raw, $\frac{1}{2}$	0.26
Wakame, dried, 8g	0.26
Sweet potatoes, $\frac{1}{2}$ cup cooked	0.27
Banana, 1 medium	0.43
Kombu, dried, 8g	0.5

Folate

Folate's major role is to help produce and maintain new cells. It also helps make our genetic keys, DNA and RNA, and prevents changes in the DNA that could lead to cancer. (*Folate* is the form of the B vitamin that occurs naturally in foods. *Folic acid* is the synthetic version found in supplements and used to fortify foods.)

MIXED GREENS

Folate is named for the Latin word *folium,* which means "leaf"—perfect because the greatest source of folate comes from leafy green vegetables.

Pregnant women, or those who have the potential to become pregnant, are advised to maintain adequate doses of folate because deficiency, especially in the first three months of pregnancy, can lead to neural-tube defects, premature birth, and/or low-birth-weight babies. Prenatal vitamins typically provide the RDA for folic acid, the synthetic form of folate.

Ironically and shockingly, recent evidence suggests that supplemental folic acid actually increases the risk for breast, colorectal, and prostate cancers, along with the risk of dying from those diseases. Studies also link folic acid supplements to an increased risk for childhood asthma and respiratory infections.

Fortunately, the natural food source (folate) does not pose any health risk as a whole food and is found in abundance in the plant world. Pregnant women and everyone else can get plenty of folate without these concerns just by eating more leafy green veggies and beans. In addition, plant-based eaters tend to have superior folate intakes and status compared to omnivores!

The RDA for folate is 400 micrograms a day for both male and female adults and 600 for pregnant and 500 for lactating women. Choose spinach, asparagus, collard greens, turnip greens, beets, lentils, pinto beans, black beans, kidney beans, and black-eyed peas for deliciously rich sources of nature-made folate.

The following table gives you the folate content found in certain foods.

Folate

Food	Folate (mcg)
Strawberries, $\frac{1}{2}$ cup	20
Tempeh, $\frac{1}{2}$ cup cooked	20
Orange juice, $\frac{1}{2}$ cup	24
Banana, 1 medium	24
Peanut butter, 2 TB.	24
Tomato juice, $\frac{1}{2}$ cup	25
Cauliflower, $\frac{1}{2}$ cup cooked	27

continues

Folate   *continued*

Food	Folate (mcg)
Tahini, 2 TB.	29
Grapefruit, 1 medium	30
Cantaloupe, 1 cup	34
Sunflower seeds, 2 TB.	40
Parsnips, $\frac{1}{2}$ cup cooked	45
Brussels sprouts, $\frac{1}{2}$ cup cooked	47
Orange, 1 medium	48
Mustard greens, $\frac{1}{2}$ cup cooked	51
Split peas, $\frac{1}{2}$ cup cooked	64
Beets, $\frac{1}{2}$ cup cooked	68
Lima beans, $\frac{1}{2}$ cup cooked	78
Avocado, raw, $\frac{1}{2}$	81
Broccoli, $\frac{1}{2}$ cup cooked	84
Turnip greens, $\frac{1}{2}$ cup cooked	85
Collard greens, $\frac{1}{2}$ cup cooked	88
Soybeans (edamame), $\frac{1}{2}$ cup cooked	100
Black-eyed peas, $\frac{1}{2}$ cup cooked	105
Kidney beans, $\frac{1}{2}$ cup cooked	115
Black beans, $\frac{1}{2}$ cup cooked	128
Spinach, $\frac{1}{2}$ cup cooked	131
Asparagus, $\frac{1}{2}$ cup cooked	134
Pinto beans, $\frac{1}{2}$ cup cooked	147
Peanuts, $\frac{1}{2}$ cup	176
Lentils, $\frac{1}{2}$ cup cooked	179

Cobalamin (Vitamin B$_{12}$)

Cobalamin, famously known as vitamin B$_{12}$, is a wildly popular topic of discussion when it comes to following a plant-based diet because it's the *only* nutrient an herbivore cannot attain directly from food or sunlight (as with vitamin D).

B$_{12}$ is made by microorganisms, bacteria, fungi, and algae. Plants and animals cannot synthesize B$_{12}$. Because animals don't wash their food before eating it, they ingest these microorganisms. They also absorb some of the B$_{12}$ produced by the bacteria in their intestines. Some plant foods may contain B$_{12}$ from contamination by those B$_{12}$-producing bacteria in the soil, but it's unlikely in developed countries due to rigorous food washing and safety practices.

Vitamin B$_{12}$ assists with several roles in the body, including red blood cell formation, neurological function, and DNA creation. It's unique because it requires intrinsic factor, made by the stomach, to be absorbed. With any stomach issues (as with pernicious anemia, an autoimmune disease) or intestinal issues, deficiency of vitamin B$_{12}$ is possible. This leads to megaloblastic anemia and neurological disorders.

You may not realize you have a deficiency until it's too late. Symptoms include decreased sensation, dementia, difficulty walking, loss of bladder or bowel control, weakness, optic atrophy, and depression. Early detection is key to preventing irreversible neurologic damage, although this can be tricky. The liver is efficient at storing vitamin B$_{12}$ for many people, and these people can go years without a deficiency. However, other people may have an undetected problem with absorption where deficiency can go on for years. It varies for each individual.

Recommended B$_{12}$ intake is 2.4 micrograms per day for adult men and women. With pregnancy, intake should be 2.6, and during lactation, 2.8 micrograms. These needs can be easily met with less than 1 tablespoon nutritional yeast or with fortified plant-based milks, cereals, and meat analogues. Or if you choose to be 100 percent unprocessed (and that deserves enormous praise!), you can safely pop a supplement to prevent deficiency.

Please note that sea vegetables, algae, and spirulina act as vitamin B$_{12}$ analogues and can actually promote deficiency. Because they look like B$_{12}$, they can attach to your B$_{12}$ receptors and take up space where real B$_{12}$ needs to be. However, these analogues have no biological activity and interfere with the absorption of the real deal.

If you don't take a B$_{12}$ supplement or use consistent amounts of fortified products (like nutritional yeast or fortified plant milks), deficiency is also probable. See Chapter 10 for more on this. Please be steadfast and cautious about your vitamin B$_{12}$ intake.

Biotin

Biotin serves as a coenzyme during the synthesis of glucose and fatty acids and for the metabolism of amino acids. Biotin deficiency is rare but will manifest as anorexia, glossitis, depression, nausea, and vomiting.

Limited data are available to form RDAs. Thus, the adequate intake for biotin is 30 micrograms per day for adults and 35 for lactating women. Excellent whole-food sources include oat bran, oatmeal, almonds, peanut butter, lentils, black-eyed peas, mushrooms, and spinach.

Pantothenic Acid

Pantothenic acid helps release energy from carbs, manufacture glucose, and synthesize and degrade fatty acids. Sources are so widespread that no reliable documented deficiencies are recorded!

Adequate intakes are 5 milligrams per day for adults. The AI increases to 6 milligrams for pregnancy and 7 milligrams during lactation. Pantothenic acid can be found in high quantities in papaya, guava, mangoes, oranges, cantaloupe, broccoli, Brussels sprouts, bell peppers, and kohlrabi.

Ascorbic Acid (Vitamin C)

Vitamin C, also known as ascorbic acid, is the other water-soluble vitamin alongside the large B-family. A very busy vitamin, C functions in varied and extensive myriad roles in the body. It helps create collagen, L-carnitine, and certain neurotransmitters. Vitamin C also acts as an antioxidant and helps in protein metabolism, immune function, and iron absorption. Deficiency leads to scurvy, which is nearly impossible on a whole-food, plant-based diet that includes plenty of fruits and vegetables.

Plant-based eaters have no problem attaining the RDA for vitamin C, which is 90 milligrams for adult men and 75 milligrams for adult women. During pregnancy, women should consume 85 milligrams per day and then 120 milligrams when nursing. Fantastic food options include papaya, guava, pineapple, bell peppers, broccoli, Brussels sprouts, cauliflower, kiwi, oranges, strawberries, cantaloupe, kohlrabi, turnip greens, and tomatoes.

The following table gives you the vitamin C content found in certain foods.

Vitamin C

Food	Vitamin C (mg)
Asparagus, $\frac{1}{2}$ cup cooked	3.5
Watermelon, $\frac{1}{2}$ cup	6
Blueberries, $\frac{1}{2}$ cup	7
Acorn squash, $\frac{1}{2}$ cup cooked	8
Spinach, $\frac{1}{2}$ cup cooked	9
Potatoes, $\frac{1}{2}$ cup cooked	10
Banana, 1 medium	10
Okra, $\frac{1}{2}$ cup cooked	13
Blackberries, $\frac{1}{2}$ cup	15
Honeydew, $\frac{1}{2}$ cup	15
Butternut squash, $\frac{1}{2}$ cup cooked	15
Edamame, $\frac{1}{2}$ cup cooked	15
Persimmon, 1 medium	16
Raspberries, $\frac{1}{2}$ cup	16
Swiss chard, $\frac{1}{2}$ cup cooked	16
Collard greens, $\frac{1}{2}$ cup cooked	17
Beet greens, $\frac{1}{2}$ cup cooked	18
Mustard greens, $\frac{1}{2}$ cup cooked	18
Turnip greens, $\frac{1}{2}$ cup cooked	20
Sweet potato, $\frac{1}{2}$ cup cooked	21
Tomato juice, $\frac{1}{2}$ cup	22
Tomato, 1 medium	23
Kale, $\frac{1}{2}$ cup cooked	26
Elderberries, $\frac{1}{2}$ cup	26
Tangerine, 1 medium	26
Cauliflower, $\frac{1}{2}$ cup cooked	27
Cabbage, $\frac{1}{2}$ cup cooked	28
Cantaloupe, $\frac{1}{2}$ cup	30

continues

Vitamin C *continued*

Food	Vitamin C (mg)
Pineapple, $\frac{1}{2}$ cup	40
Kohlrabi, $\frac{1}{2}$ cup cooked	45
Brussels sprouts, $\frac{1}{2}$ cup cooked	48
Strawberries, $\frac{1}{2}$ cup	49
Mango, 1 medium	57
Broccoli, $\frac{1}{2}$ cup cooked	58
Sweet bell pepper, $\frac{1}{2}$ cup cooked	60
Kiwi, 1 medium	64
Grapefruit, 1 medium	78
Orange, 1 medium	83
Guava, 1 medium	125
Papaya, 1 medium	188

Marvelous Minerals

Minerals are inorganic nutrients your body requires in continued supply for life, health, growth, and development. Thousands of different minerals exist in nature, but only about 21 have significant impact in your diet:

Arsenic	Molybdenum
Boron	Nickel
Calcium	Phosphorus
Chloride	Potassium
Chromium	Selenium
Copper	Silicon
Fluoride	Sodium
Iodine	Sulfur
Iron	Vanadium
Magnesium	Zinc
Manganese	

All minerals are derived from the soil and enter animals or humans via plants. And lucky for those on a plant-based diet, plants are loaded with minerals, including calcium, iron, zinc, and selenium. So the more plants you eat, the more minerals you acquire!

Macrominerals Versus Trace Elements

Minerals are divided into two groups based on whether you need a large amount (*macrominerals*) or small amount (*trace elements*, or *microminerals*).

> **DEFINITION**
>
> **Macrominerals,** also considered "bulk elements," are minerals your body needs in amounts of 100 milligrams per day or greater. **Microminerals,** or **trace elements,** are present in minute amounts in the body's tissues. For optimal health, growth, and development, you need 15 milligrams per day or less.

Recommendations for intake have been established for nine essential trace elements—chromium, copper, iodine, iron, manganese, molybdenum, selenium, zinc, and fluoride. Recommendations for five potentially essential trace elements—arsenic, boron, nickel, silicon, and vanadium—haven't yet been determined.

Because you can easily attain adequate amounts of all minerals from a whole-food, plant-based diet, I focus on the three minerals that often have absorption issues: calcium, iron, and zinc. Also, because iodine tends to be low in herbivores, I will offer some suggestions to prevent deficiency.

Calcium

Calcium is the most abundant mineral in the body—an adult human contains approximately 1,000 to 1,500 grams! Ninety-nine percent of the calcium in your body is stored in your bones and teeth, and the remaining 1 percent is throughout the rest of your body's tissues and fluids. Calcium plays an essential role in blood clotting, muscle contraction, nerve transmission, bone and tooth formation, and the secretion of hormones and enzymes.

AI recommendations for calcium in adults vary throughout the lifespan. For age 19 to 50, AI is 1,000 milligrams per day for males and females (even during pregnancy and lactation beyond the age of 19). After age 50, AI increases to 1,200 milligrams per day. Whole-plant food sources of calcium include collard greens, turnip greens, kale, broccoli, bok choy, dried figs, sesame seeds, tahini, beans, soybeans, soy nuts, and tofu.

MIXED GREENS

Bone is dynamic and is constantly breaking down and rebuilding. Even though it's seemingly always solid and hard, bone mass is turned over as much as 15 percent every year. That shows the potential of your diet to influence the strength and density of your bones throughout your lifetime. Remember, you are what you eat!

With calcium, how much you *consume* isn't necessarily the issue. What's more important is how much you *absorb*. Calcium absorption determines risk of bone fractures and osteoporosis. Many factors influence calcium absorption, including age, how much you need, how much you take in, and other compounds that accompany the calcium when you consume it. Taking effective combinations of calcium and vitamin D improves absorption.

Only minimal research on bone status in strict herbivores has been conducted so far. However, calcium is plentiful in plants, so you don't need to reach for harmful animal products to get your daily dose, which—because of their high protein, fat, cholesterol, and sodium content—wreak havoc on your arteries. If you eat your leafy greens and get plenty of exercise, you will have strong bones to last a lifetime.

The following table gives you the calcium content found in certain foods.

Calcium

Food	Calcium (mg)
Almonds, 2 TB.	24
Broccoli, ½ cup cooked	31
Lima beans, 1 cup cooked	32
Lentils, 1 cup cooked	38
Sweet potato, ½ cup cooked	45
Kale, ½ cup cooked	47
Orange, 1 medium	60
Bok choy, ½ cup cooked	79
Almond butter, 2 TB.	86
Turnip greens, ½ cup cooked	98
Tempeh, 3.5 oz.	111
Tahini, 2 TB.	128
Collard greens, ½ cup cooked	133

Food	Calcium (mg)
Sesame seeds, 2 TB.	140
Soybeans, 1 cup cooked	175
Dried figs, 1 cup	241
Soy milk, fortified, 1 cup	250 to 300
Fortified milk/juice, 1 cup	300
Tofu, calcium-set, 3.5 oz.	350 to 683

Iron

Iron is one of the most abundant metals on Earth, yet it's considered the most common nutritional deficiency worldwide! According to the World Health Organization, approximately 30 percent of the global population has iron-deficiency anemia. However, plant-based diets tend to be higher in iron than other diets. Iron is an essential component of proteins and enzymes that maintain good health, but its most important role is transporting oxygen. Almost two thirds of the iron in the body is found in hemoglobin, the protein in red blood cells that carries oxygen to the cells.

From age 19 to 50, adult men require 8 milligrams per day of iron, while women need 18 milligrams per day. After 51 years of age, the RDA decreases to 8 milligrams per day.

Diet provides two forms of iron: *heme* and *nonheme*. Heme iron is made from hemoglobin and is found in animal flesh. Nonheme iron is supplied by plants, including lentils, kidney beans, navy beans, chickpeas, pinto beans, spinach, Swiss chard, beet greens, turnip greens, pumpkin seeds, tahini, dried apricots, and blackstrap molasses.

Heme sources are absorbed better than nonheme, but this benefit may not be advantageous. More of a good thing isn't always better, and heme iron is the perfect example of when it's not. A high blood level of stored iron has been associated with increased insulin resistance and heart disease. Furthermore, iron delivered by animal products comes with saturated fat, dietary cholesterol, steroids, hormones, and antibiotics.

Iron deficiency leads to fatigue, decreased immune function, and glossitis (inflamed tongue). Loss of iron, and its resulting anemia, usually occurs due to small intestinal bleeds or kidney disease. It can also accompany certain periods of life, including age 6 months to 4 years, adolescence, pregnancy, and menstruation. Still, dietary factors impact the absorption of iron—for better and for worse.

Dietary variables that inhibit absorption of iron include phytates in whole grains and legumes, tannic acids from tea, calcium in dairy, fiber, coffee, cocoa, and some spices (such as turmeric, coriander, chilies, and tamarind). To enhance iron absorption, include a source of vitamin C with your nonheme iron-rich food. For instance, eat tomatoes with your spinach salad or strawberries in your green smoothie to maximize absorption. Other organic acids, vitamin A, and beta-carotene may also help with absorption, as does soaking and sprouting grains, beans, and seeds; leavening bread; and fermentation.

What about iron supplements, you might be wondering? They're pro-oxidative, meaning they promote oxidation. The opposite of antioxidants, they encourage free radicals to perform their mischief, thereby leading to increased risk for cancer, heart disease, aging, and other chronic diseases. Iron supplements should only be used if there's a deficiency and for as short a period as possible.

PLANT PITFALL

Phytates can block iron absorption up to 90 percent, making them significant inhibitors. Because they're primarily found in whole grains and legumes, phytates are prevalent in a plant-based diet. Fortunately, the higher the phytate content in a food, the higher the iron tends to be. Thus, consuming these products may not impact iron status as much as first thought possible. Ironically, phytates are also thought to reduce risk of various chronic diseases, including several forms of cancer!

Undoubtedly, the most telling fact about iron status in people who primarily eat a plant-based diet is that there's not much difference in incidence of iron-deficiency anemia between plant-based eaters and omnivores.

The following table gives you the iron content found in certain foods.

Iron

Food	Iron (mg)
Soy milk, ½ cup	0.55 to 0.9
Raisins, ¼ cup	0.8
Apricots, ¼ cup	0.9
Brussels sprouts, ½ cup cooked	0.9
Barley, pearled, ½ cup cooked	1.0

Food	Iron (mg)
Cashews, 2 TB.	1.0
Collard greens, $\frac{1}{2}$ cup cooked	1.1
Prunes, $\frac{1}{4}$ cup	1.2
Peas, $\frac{1}{2}$ cup cooked	1.2
Sunflower seeds, 2 TB.	1.2
Tempeh, $\frac{1}{2}$ cup	1.3
Beet greens, $\frac{1}{2}$ cup cooked	1.4
Raisins, $\frac{1}{2}$ cup	1.6
Pumpkin, $\frac{1}{2}$ cup cooked	1.7
Black beans, $\frac{1}{2}$ cup cooked	1.8
Black-eyed peas, $\frac{1}{2}$ cup cooked	2.2
Lima beans, $\frac{1}{2}$ cup cooked	2.2
Navy beans, $\frac{1}{2}$ cup cooked	2.3
Prunes, $\frac{1}{2}$ cup	2.4
Chickpeas, $\frac{1}{2}$ cup cooked	2.4
Sun-dried tomatoes, $\frac{1}{2}$ cup cooked	2.4
Pumpkin seeds, 2 TB.	2.5
Tahini, 2 TB.	2.7
Spinach, $\frac{1}{2}$ cup cooked	3.2
Lentils, $\frac{1}{2}$ cup cooked	3.3
Blackstrap molasses, 1 TB.	3.6
Nori, dried, 8g dry weight	3.7
Dark chocolate, 1 oz.	3.9
Soybeans, $\frac{1}{2}$ cup cooked	4.4
Dulse, dried, 8g dry weight	6.4
Tofu, firm, $\frac{1}{2}$ cup	6.6
Kombu, dried, 8g dry weight	22.1

Zinc

Like the other minerals, zinc is needed in many metabolic processes, including the activity of about 100 enzymes, immune function, wound healing, protein and DNA creation, and cell division. You need zinc every day because your body doesn't have a special zinc-storing system. Symptoms of deficiency include growth retardation, loss of appetite, immune impairment, hair loss, delayed wound healing, and taste abnormalities.

Adult RDA for zinc is 11 milligrams per day for males and 8 milligrams for females. However, need increases for females to 11 milligrams when pregnant and 12 milligrams during lactation. Animal products contain high doses of zinc, but you can find it in plant sources, too. Cashews, chickpeas, almonds, kidney beans, and peas are all good choices. Similar to iron, zinc absorption is inhibited and enhanced by the same nutrients.

The higher incidence of zinc deficiency in plant-based eaters is due to the fact that the absorption of zinc from plants is somewhat lower than from animal products. The Food and Nutrition Board recommends that herbivores increase their RDA by 50 percent to make up for these shortcomings.

It also recommends preparation techniques that discourage phytates from binding to zinc and increase its absorption. These techniques include soaking beans, grains, and seeds in water for several hours before cooking them and allowing them to sit after soaking until sprouts form.

You can also enhance your zinc intake by choosing leavened grain products (such as bread) instead of unleavened foods (such as crackers). Leavening partially breaks down the phytate.

The following table gives you the zinc content found in certain foods.

Zinc

Food	Zinc (mg)
Soy milk, $\frac{1}{2}$ cup	0.3
Kidney beans, $\frac{1}{2}$ cup cooked	0.8
Peas, boiled, $\frac{1}{2}$ cup	0.8
Almonds, dry roasted, 1 oz.	1.0
Chickpeas, $\frac{1}{2}$ cup cooked	1.3
Cashews, dry roasted, 1 oz.	1.6
Baked beans, canned, $\frac{1}{2}$ cup	1.7

Iodine

Iodine deficiency is a global public health concern, affecting nearly one out of every three people worldwide. Characteristics include goiter and cretinism. Brain damage occurs when iodine deficiency happens during fetal or early childhood years, so pregnant women and preschool children in low-income settings are among the high-risk populations. Recent evidence has shown a possible increased risk of deficiency in herbivores as well, especially raw followers.

Iodine is closely tied with thyroid function. When intake is low, production of thyroid hormones slows down. The RDA for children ages 1 through 4 is 90 micrograms per day and 150 micrograms per day for adults.

Iodine is hard to find in food. Because iodine content varies widely in soil, it's unreliable in plant foods. Sea vegetables can either have a lot of iodine or very little. Iodine deficiency was common in early twentieth century America until salt was iodized. Salty foods like tamari, kosher salt, and processed items don't contain iodized salt. A quarter teaspoon of commercial iodized salt contains approximately 68 micrograms, or 47 percent of the adult RDA. However, since it's not advisable to use salt, you can incorporate sea vegetables (especially dulse and kelp) into your diet and monitor for deficiency.

The following table gives you the iodine content found in certain foods.

Iodine

Food	Iodine (mcg)
Navy beans, $\frac{1}{2}$ cup cooked	32
Potato with peel, baked, 1 medium	60
Salt, iodized, 1g	77
Cod, 3 oz.	99
Sea vegetables, dried, $\frac{1}{4}$ oz.	varies up to 4,500

The Least You Need to Know

- Vitamin B_{12} isn't available from any plant-based food source. To get this vitamin, you need to take a supplement or eat fortified products.
- Vitamin D poses no more a risk for deficiency in strict herbivores than in omnivores. Although sunshine is the best source, additional supplements may be required.

- Several macrominerals and trace elements have significant impact on your diet and health, and all are available from plants.

- As an herbivore, you need to remain cognizant of the minerals calcium, iron, zinc, and iodine to ensure you meet your daily needs.

You Are What You Eat (Not What You Don't)

In This Chapter

- Fascinating facts about fiber
- Awesome antioxidants and phytochemicals
- Trans fats, MSG, and other antinutrients to avoid

When used together, two separate yet equally important components—consuming health-promoting nutrients and avoiding disease-advancing antinutrients—create the ideal diet. I've said it before: you are what you eat. What you *don't* eat is just as important to your well-being.

In this chapter, you learn more about the supernutrients that pump up your immune system by fighting on the front lines, attacking viruses, bacteria, fungi, and cancer cells every day. You also learn why ingredients such as sugar and oil do exactly the opposite in your body and put you at risk for illness and excess weight.

The Supernutrients: What to Eat

Plants come readily equipped with bounties of fibers, antioxidants, and phytonutrients. These supernutrients, abundantly provided by Mother Nature, have been found to fight the overall process of disease. Forget potions and pills … just eat plants!

Fabulous Fiber

The word *fiber* probably stirs up thoughts of powders, capsules, and prune juice, yet fiber's fabulous benefits deserve elaboration. While it's well established that fiber keeps things moving, if you will, fiber plays other health-promoting roles, from preventing cancer to managing weight. What's more, fiber is exclusively found in plants. None is found in beef, pork, chicken, fish, dairy, eggs, or other animal-derived products.

You'll remember from Chapter 2 that dietary fiber is categorized as soluble and insoluble. Soluble fiber influences positive effects on blood sugar and cholesterol levels. New research has expanded soluble fibers to include the following:

- Beta-glucans, found in oats, barley, and mushrooms, act as *prebiotics* and bind water.

- Gums and mucilages, including psyllium, carageenan, and alginates from seeds and sea vegetables, are used by the food industry to stabilize, thicken, and add texture to foods.

- Pectins, found in berries and fruits, help create jellies and jams, due to their gel-forming capabilities.

- Resistant starches come packaged in odd places, such as unripened bananas and raw potatoes, as well as in the more common legumes.

Insoluble fibers, those well known for contributing to gastrointestinal (GI) health, help by preventing constipation, *diverticulosis,* and *hemorrhoids.* Furthermore, fiber protects against colorectal cancer and possibly even gallstones, kidney stones, varicose veins, and inflammatory bowel disease (ulcerative colitis and Crohn's disease). These insoluble fibers—celluloses, hemicelluloses, and lignins—are found in whole grains, legumes, nuts, seeds, vegetables, and fruits.

Compounds named "nondigestible oligosaccharides," such as inulin and fructans found in fruits, grains, vegetables, and legumes, are multifunctional. Some act as prebiotics, while others improve intestinal health.

DEFINITION

Prebiotics are fermentable carbohydrates that encourage the growth of friendly bacteria in the GI tract. These bacteria and their by-products inhibit the growth of harmful bacteria and yeasts, reduce cancer-promoting compounds, improve absorption of minerals, and perhaps reduce food intolerances and allergies. **Diverticulosis** is a condition in which the colon has small outpouchings that may lead to inflammation (diverticulitis). **Hemorrhoids** are dilated veins in the anus or rectum, typically caused by constipation or strains due to diarrhea or pregnancy.

Moreover, fiber removes excess sex hormones from the body, especially estrogen, and eliminates heavy metals such as mercury from the GI tract. High amounts of hormones or metals hanging out in your body increase the risk for different types of cancers.

The World Health Organization and American Heart Association recommend consuming at least 25 grams fiber a day. The Institute of Medicine recommends approximately 14 grams fiber per 1,000 calories consumed for all people over the age of 1 year. Unfortunately, the average intake of fiber is approximately 15 grams or less per day! The good news is that, by eating a heavily plant-based diet, you'll naturally and effortlessly meet—and even exceed—these recommended amounts.

Popping fiber supplements or sprinkling your processed food with fiber powder isn't the same as getting that fiber from whole-food sources. Eat a variety of beans, lentils, whole grains, vegetables, and fruits every day, and you'll reap the colossal benefits associated with high fiber intakes.

Awesome Antioxidants

You've heard the term *antioxidants* bandied about in medical news, on cereal boxes, and in television ads. Still, you may not really know what's so awesome about them. It all begins with the oxygen we breathe.

Ironically (and as mentioned in Chapter 3), the oxygen we require to survive also causes aging and diseases to progress. Sounds crazy, right? During respiration (breathing), *free radicals* are formed. Free radicals are highly unstable molecules that cause oxidation to occur. Think of rust forming on metal or an apple turning brown after you cut it open and it sits out for a while—these are examples of the effects of oxidation. In the body, oxidation sets off a series of reactions that create instability and keep self-perpetuating. If these reactions aren't stopped, disease ensues.

> **DEFINITION**
>
> **Free radicals** are high-energy particles with at least one unpaired electron that go wild in the body, ricocheting around trying to match up their unpaired electrons. This causes damage and leads to heart disease, cancers, autoimmune disease, macular degeneration, impaired immunity, and accelerated aging.

Free radicals also are produced during other routine body processes, like producing energy and metabolizing drugs, and by external factors such as cigarette smoke, pollution, radiation, and chemical contamination. Essentially, it's impossible to avoid exposure to oxidation. When you exercise, you take more breaths, accelerating the formation of free radicals. This increased exposure is no excuse to forego working out (or breathing, for that matter). Enjoy a diet high in antioxidants, and the benefits of exercise far outweigh any potential damage.

This is where the beauty of antioxidants comes in. These special compounds from plants sacrifice an electron, neutralizing free radicals and stopping the process of oxidation in its tracks. Potent antioxidants include carotenoids (precursors to vitamin A), vitamin E, vitamin C, and selenium. Simply eating plenty of foods with these compounds allows you to defend yourself against the consequences of free radicals.

Carotenoids represent a family of hundreds of phytonutrients that can be converted into vitamin A—although only a few are really active. They provide a continuum of color from reds, oranges, and yellows, found in watermelon, peppers, pumpkin, papaya, tomatoes, carrots, and apricots. But they're also overshadowed by the powerful dark green color present in leafy green vegetables such as kale, spinach, and broccoli. As mentioned in Chapter 3, certain carotenoids, like lycopene in tomatoes, may be absorbed better when cooked. This is why tomato sauce more effectively reduces the risk of prostate cancer than the raw tomatoes themselves.

Vitamin E includes a family of eight antioxidants, but alpha-tocopherol, especially in food form, is the most influential on your health. A powerful force protecting cell membranes, this antioxidant is found in nuts, seeds, leafy green vegetables, and whole grains.

Vitamin C acts as an antioxidant by protecting cells from free radical damage and by helping other antioxidants, especially vitamin E, regenerate and maintain the ability to continue their work. Because vitamin C is water-soluble and is not stored in the body, it needs to be constantly replenished. On a daily basis, consume fruits and vegetables like citrus, guava, strawberries, peppers, broccoli, and Brussels sprouts to boost your vitamin C. But note: vitamin C is rapidly lost with exposure to oxygen. To minimize this effect, purchase fresh produce, store it in the refrigerator, and eat it immediately after you cut it open.

Selenium is a trace element that plays a key role in opposing free radicals. It acts as a cofactor for the enzyme called glutathione peroxidase, where it works closely with vitamin E. Excellent sources of selenium include Brazil nuts, sunflower seeds, mushrooms, whole grains, and legumes. The RDA is 55 micrograms per day for adults.

What about supplements? Unfortunately, consuming large quantities of these nutrients via supplements turns out *not* to be beneficial—and may even be harmful, really. Beta-carotene supplements, for example, increase lung cancer risk in clinical studies.

Phantastic Phytonutrients

Phytonutrients, or phytochemicals, are naturally occurring, biologically active sub-stances found in plants. (The literal translation of the Greek prefix *phyto* is "plant.") Although they're not essential for your survival, like vitamins and minerals, phytonu-trients contain potentially miraculous elements that, although meant to protect and nurture the plant they were produced for, offer those same benefits to humans. While providing color, aroma, and texture for the plants, phytonutrients also protect against predators, pests, and outside elements. In your body, their actions range from anti-inflammatory to anticancer agents, protecting you against the outside environment. (And that's just the thousands of compounds that have been discovered. Who knows how many others haven't yet come to light?)

Colorful fruits and vegetables are the record holders for all the categories of phyto-nutrients. The gold-medal winners in the phytochemical competition are dark leafy greens, cruciferous vegetables (broccoli, cauliflower, cabbage, and Brussels sprouts), blue/purple fruits (blueberries, blackberries, plums, and cherries), tomatoes, garlic, onions, citrus, flaxseeds, and soybeans. These foods are bursting with compounds like flavonoids, phenolic acids, hydroxycinnamic acids, stilbenes, lignans, carotenoids, phytosterols, and glucosinolates. Now that's a mouthful (pun intended)!

MIXED GREENS

Speaking of colors, the pigments in fruits and veggies act as phytonutrients. Chlorophyll, the most abundant pigment in plants, imparts a dark green color and is known for its powerful health-promoting effects. Therapeutically used to detoxify, heal wounds, deodorize internally, and act as an antioxidant, chloro-phyll is found in particularly high amounts in spinach, parsley, sea vegetables, and green olives.

Runners-up include tea, herbs, spices, legumes, nuts, seeds, and whole grains. Whole foods provide enhanced benefits when compared to supplements, since a powerful synergistic effect occurs in the combinations of nutrients.

So what do these special compounds actually do? Phytonutrients keep busy protect-ing your body. They help prevent cancer by blocking tumor formation, reducing cells from growing out of control, and repairing damage done to DNA. Furthermore, phytonutrients have antioxidant and anti-inflammatory actions. They boost immu-nity by fighting bacteria, viruses, and fungi. They even affect cardiovascular health by decreasing damage done to blood vessel walls, increasing blood flow, reducing blood clot formation and platelet stickiness, and decreasing blood cholesterol levels. Phytonutrients can prevent osteoporosis, macular degeneration, and cataracts.

To reap all the best health-promoting benefits, include a consistent supply of plant foods in your diet. Support your immune system with the limitless amount of powerful fibers, antioxidants, and phytochemicals naturally found in nature.

Antinutrients: What to Avoid

According to the Centers for Disease Control (CDC), in 2007 and 2008, the prevalence of obesity was 32.2 percent among adult men and 35.5 percent among adult women. What's more, in the United States, only 23.4 percent of adults eat five servings of vegetables and fruits per day, according to a self-reported survey. (And you know how those go sometimes, right? "Vegetables? Fruits? Sure, I eat them all the time! French fries and ketchup—that counts for two servings right there. Plus, I ate those with my fruit punch—there's serving number three!")

As a result, cardiovascular disease (CVD) is the major cause of death in the United States, accounting for approximately 40 percent (936,900 in 2000) of all deaths each year. Cancer is the second-leading cause of death in the United States. Approximately 1.3 million new cases of cancer are diagnosed annually. One in two males and one in three females will have a cancer diagnosis over their lifetimes. In 2002, a total of 8.7 percent of the adult population had diabetes. Moreover, about two thirds of diabetes cases go undiagnosed.

As you can see, overall our health stats are poor. Lifestyle choices are the primary factor responsible for this—chief among them, food. One of the worst things you do is assault your body every day with antinutrients: animal protein, saturated fat, hydrogenated fats, dietary cholesterol, and processed foods.

Animal Protein

For decades, experts have blamed the fat and cholesterol in animal products for their deleterious effect on the body—hence the promotion of fat-free diets, skim milk, and skinless chicken. But something surprising showed up in research in the last two decades that shifts the blame to the protein in the meat itself. Experts aren't yet teaching the protein factor for a couple reasons. Partly, this news is bad for the food industry, so they don't want the public to hear this information. In addition, all the mechanisms of how this happens are not yet perfectly understood.

However, the association between animal protein and incidence of chronic disease is strong. Animal protein is a potent carcinogen. It's the protein itself—possibly even more so than saturated fat or dietary cholesterol—that raises total body cholesterol levels, setting up the body for illness.

As I mentioned in Chapter 1, Dr. T. Colin Campbell and his associates determined the cancer-promoting effects of animal protein after a series of lab experiments. Most significantly was a study in which they injected rats with aflatoxin, a carcinogen known to cause liver cancer. Raw casein, the primary protein in dairy (at 87 percent; the rest is whey), was fed to the rats in a low-protein (5 percent) diet or a high-protein (20 percent) diet. None of the rats on the low-protein diet developed liver cancer. All the rats on the high-protein diet developed liver cancer or precancer cells. You can't get more *statistically significant* in a study: 0 to 100, all or nothing.

DEFINITION

Statistical significance is a measure of how unlikely it is that a result of a study has occurred by chance.

Additional studies using plant proteins—soy and wheat—were performed. Plant protein, even in higher amounts, did not cause cancer growth. And in further casein studies, Dr. Campbell and his colleagues turned cancer on and off simply by changing the amount of protein fed to the rats!

Dr. Campbell's comprehensive *The China Study* confirmed that populations who consume a whole-food, plant-based diet don't experience cancers or other diseases of affluence (heart disease, type 2 diabetes, and obesity). Above 10 percent of total calories from animal protein is where "the mischief begins," according to Dr. Campbell, and where disease ensues. The average intake of protein in Western societies is around 17 percent, above the danger zone. Moreover, for the majority of people, about 75 percent of that total protein intake comes from animal products. Dr. Campbell's research concludes a cancer-causing effect with a less-than-average dose of animal protein.

Although questions exist regarding this research (anytime the status quo is shaken, controversy ensues), it cannot be ignored. Dr. Campbell and his prestigious team of researchers were meticulous in their work, and critical data emerged as a result.

Saturated Fat

Saturated fat is the leading cause of high blood cholesterol, according to the American Heart Association. To combat higher cholesterol levels, it recommends an intake of less than 7 percent of total calories. The only plant sources of saturated fat are the tropical oils—coconut, palm, and palm kernel.

The health implications associated with consuming these fats include increased serum total cholesterol and LDL (the bad cholesterol), a consistently increased incidence of stroke, and poor essential fatty acids metabolism. Reducing, if not outright avoiding, tropical oils and animal products minimizes related health risks. Consuming saturated fat at all is essentially unnecessary.

Hydrogenated or Trans Fatty Acids

Hydrogenated, or trans, fats are considered the most harmful foodstuffs. These manufactured fats are used to make convenience and fast food, well, more convenient. Foods enjoy a longer shelf life, but your body is prevented from converting alpha-linolenic acid into the essential long-chain fatty acid DHA (as described in Chapter 2). Hydrogenated fats also increase your risk for heart disease.

Dietary Cholesterol

Dietary cholesterol, found in high amounts in eggs, seafood, and other animal products, was once believed to contribute to high blood cholesterol. The most current research points to the complex conversion of dietary fat and cholesterol into fat and cholesterol in your body. An increase in blood cholesterol levels is more influenced by animal protein, saturated fats, and hydrogenated fats than by dietary cholesterol.

Because only trace amounts of cholesterol are found in plant products, they're considered cholesterol-free. Furthermore, plant foods reduce blood cholesterol levels while animal products increase them. Once again, the beauty of a plant-based diet shines in the spotlight!

Oil

Oil is not a health food. All the studies linking high-fat diets to chronic disease are based on the intake of fat from animal products and vegetable oils. Oil is 100 percent fat and contains 120 calories per tablespoon. Oil is extremely nutrient-poor and calorie-rich and offers no nutritional benefits whatsoever.

MIXED GREENS

A cup of olives contains 141 calories and 4 grams fiber. A cup of olive oil, on the other hand, has 1,909 calories and 0 fiber.

Some oils contain modest amounts of vitamin E and omega-3 fatty acids, which are easily attainable from other, better sources, such as avocados, nuts, seeds, and olives. As a bonus, when you consume the whole-food sources, you also get the fiber and a multitude of other nutritious deliciousness—with fewer calories. (Although counting calories is unnecessary, eating a concentrated source of nutrient-poor calories is a surefire way of gaining weight.)

Remember that no type of oil is superior, according to the research. Coconut oil, touted for its health properties, contains about 87 percent of its total calories from saturated fat! Even the universally praised olive oil isn't healthful.

Olive oil has been hyped as a magic bullet to super heart health for years, thanks to the so-called "Mediterranean Diet." Much misinformation has been circulated since the original research—The Seven Countries Study—began in 1958. The most popular theory extrapolated from this study is that monounsaturated fat–rich olive oil decreases the risk of coronary heart disease.

Not only is this a far cry from the truth, but it's also misleading. The population that showed promising health outcomes in the original study were people living on the Greek island of Crete. In the late 1950s and 1960s, their diet consisted of fruits, vegetables, herbs, spices, beans, whole-grain breads, fish, and, yes, olive oil. It's also important to note that they were extremely active, working as farmers. The use of olive oil itself didn't cause better health profiles.

In 1997, the surviving members of the original study were reassessed. In the 30 years following, their diets became more Westernized and their physical activity drastically reduced. The Cretans' blood cholesterol levels increased, as did their weight, blood pressure, and heart disease risk.

Here are some critical points to emphasize regarding the Mediterranean Diet myth:

- Replacing saturated with monounsaturated fats is better because you're getting less saturated fat. Health benefits aren't due to the intake of the monounsaturated fats themselves.

- You don't require monounsaturated fats to stay alive. You only need the essential fats, omega-6 and omega-3 fatty acids.

- Of olive oil's total calories, 14 percent come from saturated fat.

- Olive oil didn't give the Cretans healthier hearts. Olive oil was merely one of many factors involved.

- Pouring olive oil (or any oil) on top of an unhealthy diet will *not* make you healthier.

You can get plenty of healthy fats by eating avocados, nuts, seeds, and olives instead of oils. Even leafy green vegetables contain essential fatty acids. When intact, these sources of fat maintain their other health-promoting values (phytonutrients, antioxidants, and fiber) and should be incorporated moderately into a varied, whole-food, plant-based diet.

Sodium

Sodium is an important electrolyte that regulates metabolic processes in the body. But you need only small quantities. The key word here is *small*—just 1,500 milligrams or less per day. The average 3,466 milligrams 90 percent of Americans consume daily, according to a CDC report, is excessive. Think you don't use that much? Consider this: 1 teaspoon of salt contains 2,300 milligrams sodium!

If you eat enough food to stay alive, you'll automatically consume adequate sodium for health. If you use added salt, or if you consume high-sodium foods, know this: high intakes can lead to or exacerbate hypertension, or high blood pressure. If you have high blood pressure or take medication for your blood pressure, you must maintain a sodium-sensible diet. Processed foods and restaurant dishes tend to be high in sodium. Limit these and cook with as little salt as possible.

Your palate adjusts to how much sodium you consume. The more salt you eat, the more you crave. The good news is, the less salt you eat, the less you need. Plus, dairy and processed meats are some of the highest-sodium foods. Following a plant-based diet can keep your sodium intake in check.

Sugar

Sugar is in nearly everything processed, from breads and meat-free hot dogs to candy and gum. It comes hidden in many different fancy words:

Agave	Date sugar
Barley malt	Dextrose
Beet sugar	Fructose
Brown sugar	Fruit juice concentrate
Cane syrup	Galactose
Corn syrup	High-fructose corn syrup (corn sugar)

Invert sugar

Lactose

Maltose

Organic cane sugar

Powdered or confectioners' sugar

Raw sugar

Rice syrup

Sucrose

Turbinado sugar

And that's just a sampling!

PLANT PITFALL

Three times as sweet as table sugar, agave nectar has become a hugely popular sweetener touted as a health food. Whereas table sugar is purely sucrose, which is broken down to yield half fructose and half glucose, agave can contain up to 90 percent fructose. High-fructose corn syrup is only 55 percent fructose and has become known as a health hazard. Although agave nectar brings a lower spike in blood sugar, the fructose is metabolized in the liver and may lead to elevated triglycerides, heart disease, insulin resistance, diabetes, and weight gain.

Sugar and its derivatives elevate triglycerides, blood glucose, and adrenaline. Sugar promotes cancer growth, poor cholesterol profiles, diabetes, metabolic syndrome, obesity or excess weight, gastrointestinal diseases, premature aging, depression, anxiety, cardiovascular disease, tooth and gum decay, gout, and acne. And if that weren't enough, it's physiologically addicting!

One of the best things you can do for your health (after giving up dairy and animal products, which, as an herbivore, is already crossed off the list) is to eliminate sugar. You'll find plenty of ways to indulge on a plant-based diet that will make you realize you're not missing anything. Plus, it's health-promoting to cook and bake with dates, fruits, and blackstrap molasses—but more on that later.

Artificial Sweeteners

You're born to seek out sweetness. The taste buds sensitive to the sweet flavor are located at the tip of your tongue, ready to acknowledge that sweet sensation at first lick. It's a survival mechanism. Sweet represents carbohydrates, and the most efficient form of fuel comes from those carbs. You crave sweet, so you'll seek out prime energy-producing foods first.

Evolutionarily, food has never been as accessible as it is today. In the past four or five decades, food has gone from a rare and appreciated commodity to a ubiquitous inundation of daily living. Most people in developed countries no longer eat to live but, rather, live to eat. With fast-food restaurants and convenience stores on every corner, doughnuts in every break room, and vending machines on every floor, hunting and gathering are unnecessary. Instead, messages about eating bombard your life from numerous angles.

So what's the best response to these messages? More eating, of course! Instead of worrying about where the next meal will come from, the focus has shifted to how to keep eating fast and processed foods without the health consequences. And that's how artificial sweeteners were born. And they thrive, despite the fact that no quality research indicates that they're not disease-promoting. Short-term studies funded by the sweetener manufacturers do not eliminate the fear of potential long-term damage.

The worst part about artificial sweeteners is that they trick your brain into thinking it's about to receive fuel. Yet no calories are taken in (unless you're drinking your diet soda with french fries and a large veggie cheeseburger). The only source of fuel your brain can function on is glucose (sugar). A good analogy would be filling up your car with water instead of gasoline and expecting it to function normally.

Additionally, artificial sweeteners' excessive sweetness—160 to 8,000 times the sweetness of table sugar—perpetuates the addiction to sugar more than sugar itself. For this reason, people who use artificial sweeteners have no better success at controlling their weight and health than those who eat sugar and other sweeteners.

Regardless of the *Generally Recognized As Safe* (*GRAS*) list, evidence shows the artificial sweeteners have potential to cause cancer, and no evidence to date confirms their safety.

DEFINITION

GRAS is an acronym for the phrase **Generally Recognized As Safe.** Under the Food and Drug Administration's Federal Food, Drug, and Cosmetic Act, "any substance that is intentionally added to food is considered a food additive, that is subject to premarket review and approval by the FDA, unless the substance is generally recognized, among qualified experts, as having been adequately shown to be safe under the conditions of its intended use, or unless the use of the substance is otherwise excluded from the definition of a food additive."

Artificial Colors

Artificial colors, which are possible carcinogens, have been linked to hyperactivity in children, asthma, adverse effects on the liver, and weight gain. Most of these compounds (unless specified on the package) are synthetic chemicals. They're widely available in processed foods, medications, sodas, manufactured desserts, and fast foods.

Found to be toxic to many different organs and populations, artificial colors are best avoided. Besides, whole-plant foods are gorgeously bright and colorful naturally.

Monosodium Glutamate (MSG)

Monosodium glutamate, also known as MSG, is a food additive used to create the unique taste sensation called *umami*. Meant to increase flavor intensity and improve palatability, MSG is found in Chinese cooking, as well as in processed, canned, and fast foods.

MSG acts as an *excitotoxin*, and associations have been found between MSG and incidence of Parkinson's disease, Alzheimer's disease, and Huntington's disease. Additional links have been made to asthma, headaches, heart irregularities, brain cancer, multiple sclerosis, and other serious illnesses. Children are even more susceptible to these effects because their brains are sensitive and growing, with damage possibly unseen until years later.

DEFINITION

Umami is a flavor common in Asian cooking that provides a meaty or savory type of taste. It's considered the fifth flavor after sweet, salty, sour, and bitter. **Excitotoxins** are toxic molecules, like MSG or aspartame, that stimulate nerve cells so much they're damaged or killed.

MSG is well hidden in food. Additives that *always* contain MSG include hydrolyzed protein, textured protein, plant protein extract, sodium caseinate, hydrolyzed plant protein, yeast extract, autolyzed yeast, calcium caseinate, hydrolyzed vegetable protein, and hydrolyzed oat flour. Additives that *frequently* contain MSG include malt extract, malt stock, flavoring, spices, seasoning, bouillon broth, and natural flavoring.

Hydrolyzed Vegetable Protein

Hydrolyzed vegetable protein (HVP) is a substance used in small amounts to enhance the flavor of many commercially manufactured foods such as soups, chilies, stews, dips, salad dressings, hot dogs, gravies, frozen meals, and snack foods.

HVP is created by a series of chemical processes that utilizes sulfuric acid and caustic soda (an alkalizing agent often used to make soap). The resulting brown sludge is dried, and additional MSG may be added.

This compound contains powerful brain cell toxins and several known carcinogens. HVP possibly poses an even greater danger to human health than MSG itself.

Cultivating the ideal nutrition plan is indeed a process. You need to nurture the two complementary components—the wildly nutritious elements you increase and the harmful have-nots you progressively release. Each choice on either side is progressive and optimistic and will further your fortitude in the right direction.

The Least You Need to Know

- Plants provide plenty of fiber to prevent and reverse disease by mopping up toxins and encouraging them to move along.
- While preventing the constant barrage of illness-enhancing free radicals is impossible, your best protection is frequently consuming antioxidants and phytonutrients from fresh fruits, vegetables, and other plant sources.
- Oil, sugar, and other processed foods cause toxic reactions in the body and hinder nutritional gains from whole foods.
- Basing your diet on whole foods, and avoiding the antinutrients, improves your quality of life spectacularly!

What's on the Menu?

In This Chapter

- A new set of food groups
- A bright, color-filled food guide pyramid
- Good-for-you fruits, vegetables, whole grains, and legumes
- Proper portions for your plant-based plate
- Leafy greens, the superheroes of the plant world

Dietary goals and guidelines for Americans date all the way back to 1894, when the U.S. Department of Agriculture (USDA) developed the first generation of a food composition table and guidelines. In 1916, the first daily food guide was released, illustrating the five food groups: milk and meat, cereals, vegetables and fruits, fats, and sugars. Recommendations for the use of these food groups, "How to Select Foods," appeared in 1917.

Over the next century, the USDA periodically updated and re-released food guides. These guides have progressed from 12 major food groups in 1933 to the "Basic Seven Food Guide" in 1942. In 1956, the seven were condensed to the "Basic Four" food groups—meat, dairy, fruits and vegetables, and grains—in the publication called "Essentials of an Adequate Diet." In 1979, the "Hassle-Free Guide to a Better Diet" emphasized calories and fiber, allowing sweets, fats, and alcohol to supplement the basic four food groups in moderation. Beginning in 1980, the first "Dietary Guidelines for Americans" emerged, and this report is currently updated every 5 years.

The food guide pyramid that emphasizes a hierarchy of food intake recommendations was introduced in 1992. With grains as its foundation, dairy products; meats, eggs, beans, and nuts; and fruits and vegetables were stacked on top. Sweets and fats appeared at the tip of the pyramid to represent their minimal recommended limited intake. This widely recognized pyramid was tipped over on its side in 2005, and today, you can log on to its interactive website to determine your specific food group requirements based on age, gender, weight, height, and physical activity level.

Unfortunately, politics are involved in the making of these government guidelines, thanks to lobbying and funding. Because of this, health concerns sometimes take a secondary position when determining these recommendations. However, independent entities such as Physicians Committee for Responsible Medicine (PCRM) and practicing dietitians such as myself have developed food group guidelines based strictly on health outcomes found from sound scientific research. Read on to learn about the New Four Food Groups, the Power Plate, and the Plant-Based Food Guide Pyramid.

Your New Four Food Groups

As it currently stands, the USDA's My Pyramid is divided into six categories:

- Grains
- Vegetables
- Fruits
- Oils
- Milk
- Meat and beans

However, research has proven that a diet incorporating oils, milk, and meat is high in saturated and trans fats, cholesterol, and animal protein—a significant factor in the cause of degenerative diseases.

PCRM actively works toward changing these guidelines, striving to bring healthier options to schools and the general public. Excellent resources developed by PCRM include the New Four Food Groups and the Power Plate.

Here are the New Four Food Groups:

- Vegetables
- Fruits
- Whole grains
- Legumes

Let's take a look at each in more detail.

Vegetables

Interestingly, the term *vegetable* isn't scientifically defined. Rather, it's a culinary term. The closest thing to a definition for *vegetable* is "an edible plant or part of a plant other than a seed or sweet fruit." With that definition, categorizing certain foods such as mushrooms can be tricky.

MIXED GREENS

Is corn a vegetable, fruit, or grain? Actually, it can be considered all of these. Botanically speaking, corn is a fruit. When harvested early to eat fresh, corn can be considered a vegetable. If harvested when the seeds are dry, it's classified as a grain.

The vegetable category includes the following:

Tubers are swollen underground stems that store food for the plant. They include potatoes, sweet potatoes, yams, jicama, cassava, Jerusalem artichokes, and taro.

Roots are the underground parts of plants, which, like tubers, are used for energy storage. Thereby, roots are rich in starch. Carrots, beets, turnips, rutabagas, parsnips, burdocks, and radishes are root vegetables.

Bulbs usually grow just below the surface, producing a leafy, fleshy shoot just above the ground. They usually grow in clusters or layers. Bulb vegetables include onions, leeks, garlic, and shallots.

Stems and stem shoots of the plants eaten as vegetables include celery, asparagus, kohlrabi, rhubarb, cardoon, ginger, and bamboo shoots.

Buds and flower buds are protuberances on the stems or branches of the plants. Examples are broccoli, cauliflower, Brussels sprouts, capers, globe artichokes, and cabbage.

Leaves of plants consumed as vegetables include spinach, kale, collard greens, beet greens, turnip greens, endive, lettuce, Swiss chard, watercress, arugula, purslane, rapini, radicchio, and mustard greens.

Nonsweet fruits are buds or flowers of plants that are fleshy and contain seeds. Great variation occurs with respect to appearance and composition. Vegetables in this category may include cucumbers, tomatoes, avocados, pumpkins, olives, sweet peppers, chili peppers, eggplants, breadfruits, and bitter melons.

Whole-plant sprouts are edible, germinated plant seeds usually produced by soaking seeds in a specific manner. These nutritionally dense vegetables contain high levels of vitamins, minerals, and phytochemicals. Seeds commonly sprouted and consumed are alfalfa, broccoli, chickpeas, mung beans, peas, sunflower, quinoa, clover, buckwheat, and fenugreek.

MIXED GREENS

Sprouts are superfoods. They're rich in easier-to-digest energy; bioavailable vitamins, especially B-complex, alpha-tocoherol (vitamin E), and beta-carotene (provitamin A); minerals; amino acids; proteins; enzymes; and phytochemicals because these nutrients are all necessary for a germinating plant to grow. Sprouts are easy to DIY. All you need is a clean jar, water, and some seeds, and in a few short days, you'll have sprouts.

Fungi are small, plantlike organisms that lack chlorophyll and cellulose and absorb food through their cell walls. When referring to vegetables, fungi are more commonly known as mushrooms. Lauded for their numerous health benefits, mushroom varieties include portobello, oyster, shiitake, truffle, morel, and straw.

Sea vegetables, as the name implies, come from the sea and are filled with minerals, vitamins, amino acids, and fatty acids. Included in this category are nori, dulse, kombu, and wakame.

The vegetable group consists of the most nutrient-dense food available, overflowing with vitamins, minerals, starch, fiber, phytochemicals, antioxidants, amino acids, and essential fatty acids. Veggies are also very low in calories. They provide the maximum nutritional bang for your caloric buck!

HEALTHY HINT

Cruciferous or *Brassica* vegetables are nutritional geniuses that combine vegetables from the different botanical categories. Members of the *Brassica* genus include broccoli, cauliflower, Brussels sprouts, cabbage, bok choy, collard greens, kale, mustard greens, kohlrabi, turnips, rutabaga, Chinese cabbage, arugula, horseradish, watercress, and wasabi. These veggies are unique in their known cancer-fighting properties. They are high in compounds called glucosinolates, which break down by enzymes called myrosinase into the powerful resulting indoles and isothiocyanates. They're excellent for your health—so eat lots of them!

Fruits

Colorful, sweet, and often edible, fruit is the reproductive, seed-bearing portion of a plant. Plants use fruits as a method to disperse their seeds and, using animals as the middlemen, increase proliferation.

For purposes of nutritional consideration, fruits can be divided into the following groups:

Citrus fruits are characterized by a thick rind, most of which is a bitter white pith known as albedo, covered by a thin, colored skin known as the zest. The flesh of the citrus is segmented, juicy, and acidic. Flavors range from bitter to tart to sweet. Grapefruits, lemons, limes, kumquats, oranges, and tangerines are in the citrus family.

Berries are small, juicy, antioxidant-rich fruits grown on bushes and vines. Thin-skinned berries contain many tiny seeds—so small, some are not even noticeable. Berries must be fully ripened before harvest because they won't ripen further after they're picked. Included in this category are blueberries, blackberries, raspberries, strawberries, cranberries, and currants.

Melons are members of the gourd family. The dozens of melon varieties can be divided into two general categories: sweet (or dessert) melons and watermelons. Sweet melons have a dense, fragrant flesh and a netted rind. Watermelons have a watery, crisp flesh with a thick rind. All melons are approximately 90 percent water. Included in the melon family are cantaloupe, honeydew, casaba melon, crenshaw melon, Santa Claus melon, watermelon, red seedless watermelon, and gold watermelon.

Pomes, or *tree fruits*, contain a central core with many small seeds and thin skin with firm flesh. Apples, pears, and quince are pomes.

Stone fruits, also known as drupes, are characterized by thin skin, soft flesh, and a single woody stone or pit. These fruits tend to be fragile, with a short shelf life. Included are apricots, peaches, nectarines, plums, and cherries.

Tropical fruits are native to regions around the world with hot, tropical, and subtropical terrain. Because of ample transportation, these fruits are available for consumption everywhere. The most commonly eaten tropicals are bananas, dates, kiwi, passion fruit, mango, papaya, and pineapple.

Grapes are technically berries that grow in large clusters on vines. Thanks to the wine industry, they're the largest crop in the world. With at least a dozen varieties, grapes are classified according to the color of the skin, either white or red. Not only are grapes used to make wine, but they're commonly eaten fresh or dried to make raisins. Included in the most popular varieties are Thompson seedless green grapes, Concord grapes, and red flame grapes.

Exotics include fruits from across the world that don't fit into the other categories by composition, appearance, and flavors. Guava, figs, pomegranates, prickly pears, persimmons, star fruit, and rhubarb all fall into this fascinating, flavorful category.

Fruits are healthiest when consumed fresh and as close to harvest as possible, when the nutrients are at their peak concentration. The moment a fruit is plucked, certain micronutrients begin to degrade. After fruit is cut, blended, juiced, or manipulated in any other way, oxygen exposure is maximized due to increased surface area and oxidation begins.

PLANT PITFALL

Canned fruits typically contain added syrups (sugar products), juice, and/or preservatives. Canned fruits are also subjected to high heat during the canning process. Make canned fruits your last choice for fruit options, and if you have to use them, be sure to rinse them before consuming.

Frozen fruits may be more ideal than fresh sometimes in terms of nutrient content. Fruits are usually flash-frozen, which means they're thrown in the freezer immediately after they're picked. This process slows nutrient degradation.

Dried fruits, as the name implies, are dehydrated and more concentrated sources of sugars without any of the satiating water content. Healthy treats for most, dried fruits should be limited if you're trying to watch your weight or blood sugar. Select fresh fruits instead on most occasions.

Whole Grains

Grains are a low-cost, simple staple most cultures around the world have consumed as the basis of their diets throughout history. Botanically classified as grasses that bear edible seeds, grains are also referred to as cereals. Kernels of grain are usually protected by an outer hull or husk and are composed of the germ, the endosperm, and the bran.

The germ, the smallest constituent of the grain, is the only part that contains fatty acids. The endosperm, the largest component, is high in both starch and amino acids, which is why it's the part utilized in making milled products such as flour. The bran that covers the endosperm is full of fiber and B vitamins. It (sometimes along with the germ) is removed to make refined products. To consider a grain whole, it must retain all three parts when consumed.

You can include a vast variety of whole grains in your diet. Some popular whole grains include brown rice, wild rice, barley, and oats. *Supergrains* like amaranth, quinoa, and buckwheat are excellent choices and versatile in recipes.

DEFINITION

A **supergrain** is a grain extremely high in essential amino acids, including lysine and methionine, not common in other grains. Supergrains are also exceptionally high in fiber, vitamins, and minerals.

Legumes

Legumes are plants from the pea or pod family and include all beans, peas, lentils, and peanuts. They are high in protein, fiber, vitamins, and minerals. Of the hundreds of types of beans, some are used for their edible pods, while others are used to shell for fresh or dried seeds.

In the legume category are green beans, snow peas, shelling peas, black-eyed peas, okra, all varieties of lentils, and all dried beans.

It may surprise you to find items like snow peas and okra in this category. However, the definition of a legume is a fruit or seed of any bean or pea plant consisting of a casing that splits along both sides with the seeds attached to one of those sides.

Dividing Your Plate

Now that you know all the categories and the many delicious and nutritious foods you can enjoy in each category, it's time to get some of that tasty food on your plate. But how much of what do you need? Should you get more vegetables or fruits per meal? More legumes or more grains?

When planning your meals, look at your plate—literally—and divide it into four equal sections. PCRM recommends dividing your plate into quarters for the New Four Food Groups: vegetables, fruits, whole grains, and legumes. If you see your Power Plate this way at every meal, your nutrition will automatically balance out, and you'll achieve the optimal plant-based diet.

The Power Plate

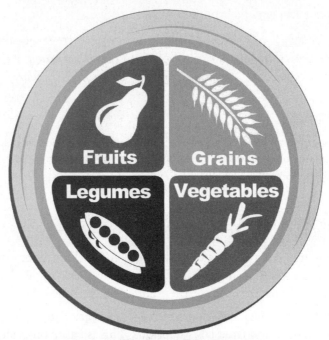

www.PowerPlate.org

The PCRM Power Plate offers a visual reminder for planning each meal by looking at what's on your plate.
(Courtesy of PCRM)

A Healthy, Plant-Based Food Guide Pyramid

As you learn more about nutrition, you're likely to come across almost as many food guide pyramids out there as you'll find diet books. However, none are true to a whole-food, plant-based nutrition plan. That's why I developed a pyramid that emphasizes nutrient density and maximizes nutritional bang for your caloric buck.

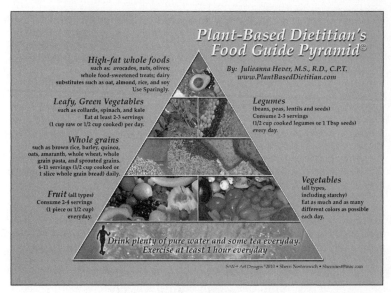

Plant-Based Dietitian's Food Guide Pyramid©
By: Julieanna Hever, M.S., R.D., C.P.T.
www.PlantBasedDietitian.com

High-fat whole foods
such as: avocados, nuts, olives;
whole food-sweetened treats; dairy
substitutes such as oat, almond, rice, and soy
Use Sparingly.

Leafy, Green Vegetables
such as collards, spinach, and kale
Eat at least 2-3 servings
(1 cup raw or 1/2 cup cooked) per day.

Legumes
(beans, peas, lentils and seeds)
Consume 2-3 servings
(1/2 cup cooked legumes or 1 Tbsp seeds)
every day.

Whole grains
such as brown rice, barley, quinoa,
oats, amaranth, whole wheat, whole
grain pasta, and sprouted grains.
6-11 servings (1/2 cup cooked or
1 slice whole grain bread) daily.

Vegetables
(all types,
including starchy)
Eat as much and as many
different colors as possible
each day.

Fruit (all types)
Consume 2-4 servings
(1 piece or 1/2 cup)
everyday.

*Drink plenty of pure water and some tea everyday.
Exercise at least 1 hour everyday*

SAN+ Art Designs ©2010 • Sherri Nestorowich • Sherrinest@mac.com

*The Plant-Based Food Guide Pyramid provides a guideline for structuring your
daily food intake.*

This pyramid is unique because fruits and vegetables are at the base (right above the
need for daily exercise and fluid consumption). This is based on evidence showing
a strong association between higher intake of fruits and vegetables and decreased
incidence of chronic disease.

The vegetable category includes carotenoid-rich and starchy vegetables. Carotenoid-
rich vegetables are high in antioxidants that protect cells from the damaging effects
of free radicals, provide a source of vitamin A, enhance immune function, and help
the reproductive system function. Specifically, this category includes carrots, greens,
sweet potatoes, tomatoes, pumpkin, and bell peppers. The starches are rich sources of
complex carbs and fiber, and include potatoes, squash, and corn.

Fruits contribute vitamin A, vitamin C, some B vitamins, and some minerals. Dried
fruits may contain iron. This section contains all whole fresh fruits and frozen fruits—
the priority and majority of fruit consumption—as well as dried fruits, whole fruit
juices, and canned fruits (in order of health-promoting capacity).

A separate category is included for leafy green vegetables. Leafy greens are chock-full
of macro- and micronutrients, including calcium; fiber; folate; vitamins C, B_6, B_2,

and E; potassium; manganese; magnesium; and phytochemicals such as lutein, beta-cryptoxanthin, zeaxanthin, and beta-carotene. This category of vegetables includes kale, collard greens, spinach, mustard greens, beet greens, turnip greens, romaine lettuce, bok choy, Swiss chard, rainbow chard, Brussels sprouts, sea vegetables, broccoli, and napa cabbage.

Moving on up the pyramid, we find that whole grains are the backbone of the plant-based diet because they contribute calories, fiber, protein, iron, B vitamins, and trace nutrients. This category includes whole-grain breads, cereals (such as oats), bulgur, millet, quinoa, buckwheat, whole-grain pasta, barley, brown rice, polenta, wheat berries, popcorn, amaranth, corn, and sprouted tortillas.

Legumes provide a supporting role in the diet. They're used extensively in international cuisines and provide protein, fiber, iron, calcium, zinc, and selenium. Legumes include cooked and dried beans (adzuki beans, anasazi beans, black beans, black-eyed peas, cannellini beans, chickpeas, fava beans, Great Northern beans, kidney beans, lima beans, navy beans, pinto beans, soybeans), lentils, peas, split peas, and soy products (tempeh, tofu).

At the top of the pyramid is a category for high-fat whole foods, dairy substitutes, and whole-food sweetened treats. High-fat whole foods refer to olives, avocados, nuts, and seeds. These foods provide omega-3 fatty acids, monounsaturated fatty acids, fiber, protein, fat, iron, calcium, and trace minerals. All of these items should be used sparingly—even less if weight loss is a goal or when heart disease, diabetes, high cholesterol, or other metabolic conditions have been diagnosed.

Overall, this pyramid is intended for use as a guideline. Perfecting the serving sizes is not necessary. Look at it as a way of proportioning out what a day's worth of food should look like. The foods closer to the bottom should be a mainstay or foundation of intake, and those near the top are to be used as support.

Let Thy Greens Be Thy Medicine ...

Emphasizing these truly magical foods is warranted because they're genuinely like nature's medicine. No other food group is as nutrient-dense as leafy green vegetables. Here are some of the reasons greens are the superheroes of the plant-based world:

- Because leafy greens are so low in calories and high in fiber, they're ideal for weight management.

- They're cancer-fighting powerhouses.

- Atherosclerosis, the process of clogging arteries, is hindered by leafy greens.

- Leafy green intake is associated with a lower risk of type 2 diabetes.

- The carotenoids help boost immunity.

- Leafy greens are excellent for your bones because they're higher in calcium than any other whole-plant food.

Every disease process can be ameliorated in some way by a consistent supply of leafy green vegetables. Because of their strong ability to heal and prevent, treating your body to a constant stream of greens like spinach, kale, collard greens, and all the others previously mentioned will do it good. You can do this easily by making green smoothies and adding leafy greens to soups, pasta dishes, stews, salads, and virtually any recipe you make. Ask for side dishes of steamed greens when eating out, and order a salad as an appetizer or as the main dish.

Greens range from neutral in taste to bitter, so you can match them with what you're eating. For green smoothies, which are typically fruit-sweetened, use the milder greens, such as dandelion greens, spinach, and kale. If you prefer the bitter, pungent flavors, try dishes using arugula or mustard greens.

HEALTHY HINT

A fabulous way to ensure you get plenty of green leafies every day is to make a green smoothie for breakfast every morning (see Chapter 20 for some recipes). You can really pack a punch by putting some greens along with frozen fruit and a liquid into a blender, and voilà! A perfectly nutrient-dense meal that will boost energy, keep you full for hours, and start your day off right.

With so many different varieties and tastes, you can experiment to see which ones you prefer to eat and in what ways. Just be sure to eat them as often as possible to boost and protect your health!

The Least You Need to Know

- The focus of your plant-based diet should be on the New Four Food Groups: vegetables, fruits, whole grains, and legumes. Visualize your plate divided into quarters for serving these foods in adequate portions.

- A huge variety of whole-plant foods can tempt your creativity and easily keep your nutrition sound.

- The Plant-Based Food Guide Pyramid is a useful tool to help guide your daily food choices.

- Incorporate leafy green vegetables into your day as often as possible to benefit your health in every way possible.

Living a Plant-Based Life

Confusion and controversy abound when it comes to nutrition. Unfortunately, when guidelines get complicated, the result is often a level of detachment. And really, why bother trying so hard when even the experts disagree? Instead of trying to deconstruct the details, let's keep it simple and stick to the basics.

In Part 2, you learn how to listen to your body's cues and focus on the quality of the food you eat instead of getting caught up in the numbers. I also demystify the most controversial claims in the plant-based world and show you how to make shopping for food fun and uncomplicated.

A health-promoting lifestyle would be incomplete without including exercise. That's why I added a chapter full of all the information you need to find and commit to the perfect workout program for your lifestyle.

Finally, do you really need to be popping supplements to achieve and maintain optimum health? Find out all the facts about supplementing in Chapter 10.

Stop Counting, and Start Eating

In This Chapter

- Analyzing nutrition for quality versus quantity
- Defining nutrient density
- Getting to know yourself from the inside out

We've lost sight of the meaning of health. Health isn't merely the absence of disease; it's so much more. Our bodies are ingeniously designed to have boundless energy, resist illness, live well into our 90s without pain or disease, and die quietly in our sleep at a ripe, old age. Yet more people than ever are sick, overweight, and in pain. Health care has become little more than treating symptoms with chemistry experiments (polymedications) and procedures. It's time to see the forest instead of the trees, to shift the focus to prevention instead of treatment.

You eat at least three times a day, every day, and your food is the direct link from the outer environment into your body. That means you literally are what you eat. More specifically, you are what you absorb. Did you know that your GI tract plays a significant role in your immune system? Ironically, your body knows precisely what it needs not only to be absent of disease, but to flourish and be productive. Learning to hone in on and listen to the cues your body's sending may provide you with the knowledge you need to take your health to the next level.

The Downside of Our Obsession with Numbers

We've become obsessed with numbers. How much do you weigh? How much *should* you weigh? How many calories should you eat? What percentage of carbs is ideal? How many ounces should you eat? How many milligrams of calcium should you take to prevent osteoporosis? And on and on.

Ironically, the more we count, the worse our health is becoming. Something's wrong with this picture.

The thousands of diet books on bookstore shelves today promise to make you healthier, leaner, and fitter as long as you follow the directions precisely. Unfortunately, the onslaught of new formulas and prescriptions has resulted in mass confusion and nutrition information chaos. As a nutrition counselor, my job description has been redefined as "nutrition myth-debunker." Instead of teaching from scratch, my job has transitioned toward explaining why what's out there is false or misleading. One day, one type of fat is good for you and another is bad. The following day, avoiding fat entirely is headline news. With all these conflicting theories, it's no wonder people are having such a hard time figuring it all out.

In addition to the lack of clarity regarding how best to eat, you'll experience the other side of health care. Physicians mostly treat symptoms by prescribing medication. In medical school, students receive minimal education about nutrition; what they do learn is usually based on correcting nutrient deficiencies. If, for example, a patient comes in with a goiter, she or he has an iodine deficiency and needs a prescription for iodine. Or if a child presents signs of rickets, he or she is deficient in vitamin D and needs vitamin D supplements.

This is isolated, microscopic, and reductionist health care. To treat a patient, a physician needs to examine the whole patient. More holistic questions need to be asked. Why is the patient struggling with weight? Why does the patient have high cholesterol? The *source* of the problem needs to be established and must become the focus of the treatment protocol.

When was the last time your doctor asked about your diet or exercise habits? This is rare, yet this is how health needs to be addressed to solve the health-care crisis.

We've strayed from the Hippocrates style of medicine: "Let thy food be thy medicine and thy medicine be thy food." Dr. Caldwell Esselstyn, author of *Prevent and Reverse Heart Disease*, said in an interview recently that this is the first time since Hippocrates that physicians don't tell people the cause of their disease.

The Best Nutrient Bang for Your Caloric Buck

You can consume only so much food in a day. Some people can eat more than others, and of course, some *should* be eating more than others. Everyone has a unique metabolism, requiring different amounts of food to support body weight, activity level, and hunger cues. Of those total calories needed per day, the majority need to come from nutrient-dense foods.

Unfortunately, this is not the modus operandi of most people. For example, the USDA Food Guide Pyramid allows 12 teaspoons of added sugars per day on a moderate 2,200-calorie diet. But the average consumer eats closer to 31 teaspoons per day. Considering 1 teaspoon sugar equals 4 grams and 16 calories, that's nearly 500 extra health-degrading, nutrient-void calories each day!

> **MIXED GREENS**
>
> In the past three decades, consumption of processed fats and sugars has continuously increased, especially from products like high-fructose corn syrup, vegetable oils, shortening, heavy cream, and refined flours. Approximately one third of added sugar intake comes from nondiet soda, and 10 percent from other types of fruit drinks (not 100 percent fruit).

Eating empty calories—or replacing room in your stomach with nutrient-poor foods—wastes an opportunity to nourish your body. Foods that come without fiber, antioxidants, vitamins, minerals, and phytonutrients are either just plain calories at best or harmful at worst. "Foods" stripped of nutrients not only neglect to provide nutrition, but they also act as antinutrients, as defined in Chapter 4.

Make Every Bite Count

Nutrient density is the ratio of nutrients per calorie (or energy content). It can also be thought of as the amount of micronutrients per macronutrients. The goal is achieving the most nutritional bang for your buck and making every bite count as much as possible.

Joel Fuhrman, M.D., believes food addiction and overeating are promoted by micronutrient inadequacy and recommends a diet rich in plant-derived micronutrients. His findings demonstrate that eating more foods higher in micronutrients is critically important for weight loss because it derails food cravings, addictions, and overeating behavior. His health equation $H = N \div C$ (where H equals healthy life expectancy,

N is nutrients, and C is calories) suggests that your late-life health is proportional to your nutrient-per-calorie intake throughout your lifetime. Eating foods with more nutrients per calorie leads to better health and enhanced protection against the diseases common in later life.

Dr. Fuhrman is also the developer of ANDI, or the Aggregate Nutrient Density Index. ANDI classifies foods based on their concentration of important nutrients. Dr. Fuhrman recommends consuming 90 percent of total calories from whole, natural plant foods, or those foods richest in micronutrients with anticancer benefits: vitamins, minerals, and phytochemicals.

The nutrients that determine foods with the highest ANDI scores include calcium, carotenoids (beta-carotene, alpha-carotene, lutein, and zeaxanthin), lycopene, fiber, folate, glucosinolates, iron, magnesium, niacin, selenium, vitamin B_1 (thiamin), vitamin B_2 (riboflavin), vitamin B_6, vitamin B_{12}, vitamin C, vitamin E, zinc, and ORAC score × 2. (Oxygen Radical Absorbance Capacity is a method of measuring the antioxidant or radical-scavenging capacity of foods.)

MIXED GREENS

Kale and collard greens received a perfect ANDI score of 1,000. Cola received a score of 1.

Foods that meet the nutrient-dense criteria include leafy green vegetables, cruciferous vegetables, berries, onions, garlic, mushrooms, orange foods (like carrots, cantaloupe, yams, and oranges), lentils, flaxseeds, and beans.

To prevent—and even reverse—disease, the majority of your food choices should be nutrient-dense. Concentrate on a variety of colors, as the hues represent the different, superhealthy phytonutrients.

Rethink Refined Food

Now that you know the reasons whole-plant foods are your best friends when it comes to nutrition, it stands to reason that their polar opposites, *refined foods*, need to be left by the wayside. Besides being pumped up with antinutrients (see Chapter 4), they typically exemplify a nutritional void—empty calories without fiber or micronutrients.

DEFINITION

Refined foods are stripped of their intact parts, as when whole grains have their bran and/or germ removed, leaving only the endosperm. Think white flour and white rice. Refined products can also be called *polished* or *processed*.

The composition of refined foods can provide a possible explanation for overeating. These products have high concentrations of sugar and other refined sweeteners, refined carbohydrates, fat, salt, and caffeine—all addictive substances. Many people can't regulate their consumption of such foods. This loss of control could account for the global epidemic of obesity and other metabolic disorders. Addiction to refined foods conforms to the diagnostic criteria for substance use disorders.

Foods that can be considered refined include the vast majority (or totality) of what can be bought at a fast-food restaurant; foods that come packaged with ingredients you don't recognize or with more than three unrecognizable ingredients; fried foods; frozen meals; foods that appear oily, salty, or sugary; most foods from a vending machine; packaged cookies, cakes, crackers, and candies; and foods such as flour, sugar, oil, margarine, and soda.

In addition to the saturated and hydrogenated fat, sodium, sugar and/or artificial sweeteners and colors, MSG, and HVP, you may find plenty of other not-so-goodies in your refined—or processed—food. These include but are not limited to preservatives, artificial flavors, thickeners, shelf-stabilizers, high-fructose corn syrup, genetically modified organisms (GMOs), sugar alcohols, nitrites and nitrates, and butylated hydroxyanisole.

MIXED GREENS

Processed foods can technically be anything that originally comes from nature but is then manipulated via cooking, cutting, juicing, blending, or any other physical maneuver that changes its form or exposes it to oxygen or other elements. The term is typically used interchangeably with *refined foods;* however, healthy foods can be processed—green smoothies, for instance. So processed doesn't *always* mean harmful.

You can avoid the harmful effects of these unnatural and health-demising chemicals by sticking to a whole-food, plant-based diet. A good rule of thumb is that if you can't pronounce it, don't eat it! And if you can't find it living freely in nature, avoid it!

Listening to Your Internal Signals

You, like all humans, have a built-in monitoring system designed to alert you when you're hungry, full, tired, or in danger. But somehow, we've learned to quiet and suppress these signals in order to make deadlines, satisfy cravings, stifle emotions, deal with stress, and so on. The connection to true innate physiological needs is lost in most people. Yet your body knows itself better than anyone else does, so listen to it!

You might be wondering why it's important to reconnect with those signals. Isn't it better to stay on time and keep up with the chaos? No. Not if you want to function at peak performance. You need to relearn to fuel yourself with the right foods, in the right way.

The number obsession I wrote about earlier in this chapter illustrates our disregard for our body's internal cues. If you're counting how many calories you've eaten, you'll choose what's for dinner based on calories rather than your level of hunger. Your body deserves to be heard. Tuning in to the cues your body's sending you makes attaining and maintaining an ideal weight effortless. Plus, your health will be enhanced tremendously.

> **HEALTHY HINT**
>
> Are you eating emotionally? If you are, make a list of activities you can do to distract yourself from stress, boredom, or other emotionally charged reasons. If stress is the trigger, take a walk, play with your pet, or take a soothing bath. If you're bored, call a friend, exercise, go window shopping, or browse the Internet for plant-based news, recipes, or health articles.

The Metabolism Myth

A common theory fitness and health professionals teach is to eat frequently throughout the day to boost metabolism. This method is based on the idea that keeping your body digesting is a way to prevent overeating and maintain energy, making you lean and healthy. But what if I told you this thinking puts you at a disadvantage?

Throughout history, scientific experiments have confirmed that animals live longer when put on a calorie-restricted diet. The research has consistently shown that slimmer people tend to be healthier overall. What can we extrapolate from these data? The slower your overall metabolism, the slower you age. This may sound shocking and, possibly, confusing. However, read on to understand the science supporting this principle.

Logic would dictate that the more food you eat, the harder and more frequently your body has to digest and assimilate these nutrients. Digestion and absorption require approximately 10 percent of total body energy—energy pulled from basic metabolic functions. In other words, the less time your body works on digestion, the more time it focuses on repair, healing, and other metabolic processes necessary to sustain health.

Calorie restriction is one of the most potent findings in slowing the process of aging and disease. The message contradicts common teachings and societal norms. Ultimately, to decrease your risk of most diseases and to increase your lifespan, you must eat a diet based in whole-plant foods.

Additionally, you must eat only as much as necessary. That means eating only when hungry and stopping before feeling overfull. You might benefit from eating at an early hour each night. Then you complete digestion before sleep, which gives your body the whole night to heal, recover, and fight disease processes.

Also, instead of eating just because it's breakfast time or because others are eating, wait until your body truly feels hunger. Then provide nutritious, whole-plant foods to your prepared digestive system.

How to Hear Hunger

Inner mechanisms for regulating eating are long lost in most people and need to be relearned. Abandon any preexisting rules you've set in your mind.

Are any of these commonly touted ideas part of your mind-set?

- Eat breakfast as soon as possible, even if you're not hungry.
- Eat every three or four hours to prevent hunger from kicking in.
- Eat three square meals and two snacks each day.
- Finish your meal before you have dessert.
- Eat 4 ounces protein, 1 cup starch, and 1 cup vegetables at every meal.
- For every pound of your ideal body weight, eat 10 calories per day.

What all these rules have in common is their disconnect from your body's needs. Your nutrient requirements are impacted by your daily life. When you're sick or fighting illness, your body needs to focus on immune function. Digestion and absorption will divert energy away from your immune system, so eating less is better. Plus, you're probably naturally less hungry when you're under the weather, so listen to your body.

Conversely, a great workout causes your body to send larger, louder hunger signals. Your body needs to replenish energy stores and to rebuild and repair the microdamage to the muscles and bones during your workout. Your body wants permission to ignore the rules. It knows when it needs to eat, how much it needs, and when it's done eating for that meal.

You can gauge your hunger on a scale from 0 to 10: 0 means you're starving, and 10 means Thanksgiving-full. Optimally, you should eat starting at 1 or 2 and stop at about 6 or 7. Eat only when you feel true hunger—but *not* at the point that you feel weak, shaky, headache-y, or ill—and stop when you feel comfortably satiated.

> **PLANT PITFALL**
>
> If you're not hungry enough to eat an apple, you're probably not really hungry.

Like anything, practice makes perfect. If you tune in, your body's natural signals will get louder and brighter and, ultimately, impossible to miss. Start every day with an open mind, and allow your body to become hungry before that first meal. Then indulge your hunger with a colorful, phytochemical festivity to make your cells sing blissfully. Eat until you feel good and then move along with the next part of your day. You may not feel hungry again for several hours, depending on how much exercise and daily activity you engage in, how much your individual body needs to stay at its current weight, and how much you slept the night before.

Because so many variables come into play, you can see why it's senseless to follow arbitrary rules. Bask in your uniqueness. Honor it, and respect your individuality. Your body will thank you by maintaining superlative weight and health.

Quality Over Quantity

Quality of food needs to dominate over quantity. Clearly, counting and quantifying is ineffective. Choosing from whole-plant foods every time your body tells you it's hungry nourishes your cells, provides satiety, and sustains your disease-fighting mechanisms. You literally empower your immune system to fight off foreign invaders, slow the aging process, and maintain a lean physique by choosing nutrient-dense sources of fuel. It really is that simple.

The Least You Need to Know

- Counting, weighing, measuring, and obsessing won't make you healthy—and could be detrimental to your well-being.
- Hippocrates was spot-on when he stated, "Let thy food be thy medicine, and thy medicine be thy food."
- Maximize your health by selecting whole, nutrient-dense plant foods that remain as close to nature as possible.
- Your body knows what it needs. Listen to its hunger cues to achieve your best health.

Controversy Clarified

In This Chapter

- Why dairy *doesn't* do a body good
- Building strong bones to last a lifetime
- Dispelling soy safety rumors
- A closer look at genetically modified organisms
- Benefits and concerns of a raw diet

Nutrition is one of the most controversial and dynamic sciences. Information changes daily, and experts disagree on how to interpret that information. In this chapter, I break down the most common controversial nutrition issues and provide you with the most up-to-date wisdom on each topic.

The Dairy Dilemma

One of the most brilliant marketing campaigns ever to saturate popular culture comes from the dairy industry. From posters and handouts given to school children to star-studded television and magazine ads, we're officially convinced a healthy diet must include dairy products. Government guidelines recommend two or three servings of dairy products per day. Is it because calcium is best delivered by dairy? Or is it because the lobbying and funding of the dairy industry have tremendous influence?

About 70 percent of the world population has difficulty digesting dairy products due to a condition called *lactose intolerance*. Humans aren't genetically programmed to consume dairy. We're the only species that drinks the milk of another species, consuming milk after weaning. Currently, some dietitians and physicians encourage lactase enzymes or other medications so patients can push past symptoms and still consume dairy. If your body tells you "no," you might want to pay attention. Besides, plenty of calcium sources in the plant kingdom don't cause discomfort when consumed.

> **DEFINITION**
>
> **Lactose intolerance** is the inability to digest lactose, the sugar component of milk, due to the body's failure to produce the enzyme lactase. Gastrointestinal symptoms vary from mild to extreme and can include gas, bloating, cramps, diarrhea, and extreme pain.

In population studies, cultures that consume the highest amounts of calcium and dairy products also have the highest incidence of osteoporosis and bone fractures. Conversely, societies that exclude dairy products from their diets experience much lower rates of bone fracture. If what we're told about drinking milk is true, how could this be possible?

The Real Effect of Dairy on the Bones

Dairy does indeed contain high amounts of calcium, which is an important mineral for bone metabolism. However, it also contains high amounts of animal protein (and sodium in cheese), which causes increased amounts of calcium to be excreted in the urine. The resulting acid environment formed in the blood—a condition known as metabolic acidosis—is thought to be caused by excessive intakes of animal protein, especially when accompanied by low intakes of fruits and vegetables. Calcium and phosphorus may be leached from your bones, sent into your bloodstream to buffer the acid, and ultimately excreted via urine.

However, this explanation is being questioned based on some recent evidence that, perhaps, the calcium and protein in the dairy may overcompensate for this effect. Because many mechanisms come into play and bone metabolism is a very complex series of processes, scientists are not in agreement on exactly how dairy impacts bone health. Regardless of whether dairy negatively impacts your bones, the other well-established harmful effects justify the recommendation of minimizing—if not eliminating—dairy products from your diet.

Optimizing Bone Density

Bone health is a complex and multifactorial process. Bone mass accumulates most during the first couple decades of life. The more bone gained during this period, the less risk of osteoporosis you face later in life. Unfortunately, this critical window closes before most young people even hear the word *osteoporosis*. If you did know to focus on bone-building during your teenage years, what would you actually do? The same things you should do at any age to optimize bone density.

MIXED GREENS

Developing bones require sufficient amounts of many nutrients. Calcium has received the most attention because of its great mass present in the adult skeleton: more than 1,400 grams in males and 1,200 grams in females.

Interestingly, the number-one factor for improving and maintaining bone health isn't at all food related: the best way to build bone is to perform weight-bearing exercise regularly. Resistance exercise improves bone density more than any dietary factor. Lift weights, walk, jog, jump, or do callisthenic exercises at least three or four times a week to keep your bones, muscles, tendons, and ligaments strong and pliable.

Nutritional recommendations include eating adequate amounts of fruits and vegetables, cutting out dairy, maintaining optimal vitamin D levels, and consuming plant-based sources of calcium every day.

Vitamin D plays an important role in bone mineralization, working with calcium to break down old bone cells and build up new ones. You can be sure you're getting enough vitamin D with a simple blood test. Remember from Chapter 3 that the ideal result of the 25-hydroxyvitamin D test is at least 50 ng/mL.

If you're not there (like the vast majority of the population), try spending 15 to 20 minutes in the sun three times a week. Apply sunscreen only to your face, exposing your arms, legs, and whatever else you can reveal without offending the neighbors. The sun is the best source for vitamin D. Sun-derived D stays in the body the longest, and you can't get vitamin D toxicity from the sun. The sun offers other health benefits—it releases feel-good endorphins and regulates your circadian rhythm.

If after a few weeks you're still testing low, consider supplementing with vitamin D_2. You can safely start out with 1,000 to 2,000 IU per day. If you're deficient, taking

5,000 to 6,000 IU per day for 2 or 3 months is safe. Please check your blood levels before supplementing, and ask your physician to monitor and help you reach your goals.

HEALTHY HINT

Vitamin D_2, ergocalciferol, is the vegan version, while vitamin D_3, cholecalciferol, is derived from animals.

Plant Sources of Calcium

Calcium is plentiful in the plant-based world. Best of all, plant sources of calcium are well absorbed, with only positive effects on your health.

Once again, magical leafy green veggies rank high on the list. Kale, collard greens, turnip greens, and cabbage contain high quantities of absorbable calcium. Fortified plant milks and juices, tofu (set in calcium), broccoli, unhulled sesame seeds, tahini, and blackstrap molasses also are excellent plant sources of calcium and should be considered part of a nutritious daily diet.

Other Problems with Dairy

Dairy increases growth hormones in your blood. Insulin-like growth factor-1 (IGF-1) helps a baby calf double its birth weight in less than 2 months—more than three times faster than a human infant does. In humans, IGF-1 causes undesirable growth, and a high level of IGF-1 is a known risk factor for cancer. In fact, IGF-1 increases prostate cancer risk by more than five times!

Early dairy consumption has been linked to type 1 diabetes, the autoimmune type typically diagnosed in childhood. Type 1 diabetes occurs when the immune system attacks pancreas cells, permanently destroying the pancreas's ability to produce insulin. Once this diagnosis is made, the person must take insulin for the rest of his or her life. Type 1 diabetics also are at increased risk for other chronic conditions later, like cardiovascular disease. Risk of type 1 diabetes increases by 11 to 13 times in children who have early exposure to cow's milk.

Moreover, dairy is abundant in dietary cholesterol and saturated fat. Even skim milk contains cholesterol: 1 cup contains 5 milligrams versus 25 milligrams in whole milk, which also has 5 grams saturated fat. A cup of cheddar cheese (easily found on a large piece of pizza) provides a whopping 139 milligrams cholesterol, 28 grams saturated fat, and 532 calories.

Milk products are inundated with steroids and hormones (both naturally occurring and production-induced) that are linked to cancer and other potential health problems. Genetically engineered growth hormones, insulin-like growth factor-1, estradiol, progesterone, and testosterone fill dairy products to the brim. Even organic "hormone-free" dairy products contain hormones, just not necessarily at the same levels.

Also in your chemical cocktail lies antibiotic residues, pesticides, herbicides, fungicides, veterinary drugs, fertilizers, synthetic preservatives, and additives. Surprisingly, many studies find little difference between levels of the aforementioned compounds in organic dairy when compared to conventional. So just because you pay more for the "organic" label doesn't mean you're getting a safe, toxin-free product. Microbiological contaminants (think bacteria, viruses, parasites, and mycotoxins) can also find their way into your dairy products and other animal products.

Dairy consumption may cause iron deficiency because it inhibits absorption. (This explains the recommendation that infants under 1 year of age not drink cow's milk.)

MIXED GREENS

White blood cells, or pus, are found in dairy products due to the infections the cows regularly acquire during the unnaturally high processing demands.

Ultimately, dairy does more damage than good. If you feel you can't give up dairy (especially cheese), blame the casein; this protein causes the production of the same feel-good effects as opiate drugs. When consumed, casein converts into casomorphins—nature's way to ensure an infant will return to the breast for milk. In cheese, the protein (mostly casein) is much more concentrated along with the fat and sodium content than in milk. Together, you have a powerfully addictive mixture. In fact, PCRM's Dr. Neal Barnard was able to use naloxone—an opiate-blocker medication used to counteract heroin and morphine overdoses—to cut cravings for cheese and other addicting foods (meat, sugar, and chocolate). Cut out dairy, and your cravings will go away in about 3 weeks.

Soy Confusing

Soy has been a favorite staple of plant-based eaters for decades. Nutritionally, soy packs a powerful punch: more protein than most other legumes, ample fiber, omega-3 fatty acids, calcium, and iron. Soy also supplies health-promoting phytonutrients like isoflavones that reduce cholesterol levels and cancer risk.

As a bean, soy can be eaten from the pod when cooked, fermented into miso paste or tempeh, curdled into tofu, or processed into milk or various other products. As an ingredient, processed soy is found in hundreds of products on the market today, including faux meats and baby formulas. It's available as textured vegetable protein, hydrolyzed vegetable protein, soy lecithin, soy flour, isolated soy protein, defatted soy flour, and soy protein concentrate.

Is Soy Safe?

Controversy rages when it comes to soy. Due to the wealth of nutrients and potential health claims soy has to offer, there has been an intensified explosion of studies. Varying conclusions make it hard to read between the lines and know what to believe. Let's break down some of the recent issues.

Does soy promote or prevent hormone-sensitive cancers (breast and prostate)? The isoflavones in soy act as *phytoestrogens*, but it's unknown whether these stimulate or inhibit the growth of cancer cells. Of the many studies available, few were done with humans. Furthermore, an isolated part of the soy (mostly the isoflavones) is used instead of the intact bean. Consuming foods in their whole forms is beneficial. In Asian countries, where soy has been eaten as a condiment for centuries, the breast and prostate cancer rates are four to six times lower than those in the West. More research is needed before conclusions can be made on soy with respect to cancer.

Another soy concern is its possible interference with thyroid function. Soy has been reported to cause *goiters*, hypothyroidism, and thyroid cancer. But adequate intake of *iodine* reverses any goiter-causing effect of soy in a healthy person. Plant sources include iodized salt, sea vegetables, and plants grown in iodine-rich soil. Additionally, population studies have shown a protective effect of soy on thyroid cancer.

DEFINITION

Phytoestrogens are plant compounds, similar to the hormone estrogen, that look and act like estrogen in the body. A **goiter** is an abnormally enlarged thyroid gland most commonly due to iodine deficiency in the diet, but it can also occur with other thyroid disease. **Iodine** is a trace mineral required in the diet to help with metabolism.

The media have propagated concerns about soy's effect on hormones. You may have heard how soy consumption decreases fertility or gives a male "man-boobs." But no solid evidence supports these assertions.

Similarly, fears circulated that soy-based infant formulas led to problems with sexual development, brain function, immunity, and future reproduction. No conclusive evidence supports these claims, either. Most experts are confident in recommending soy-based formulas.

Soy can be part of a balanced plant-based diet. For safe soy consumption ...

- Consume soy from whole-food or minimally processed sources—soybeans, tofu, tempeh, miso, soybean sprouts, and soy milk.

- Use soy in moderation—less than 3 servings per day, where a serving is 1 cup soy milk or $\frac{1}{2}$ cup soybeans, tofu, or tempeh.

- Avoid processed soy products, like soy protein isolates (found in protein drinks and bars, meat analogues, cereals, meal replacement products, and other processed items).

- Consume only organic or genetically modified organism–free soy products.

Are Genetically Modified Organisms Okay?

In the age of biotechnology, scientists have found ways of manipulating the genes of organisms. Genetically modified organisms, or GMOs, are the results of the permanent alterations of the inherent blueprints of seeds. By doing this, desired traits in plants are enhanced, providing promise for solutions to world hunger, environmental issues, and human health. But is this too good to be true?

Arguments for the use of GMOs include better resistance to stress from weather and pest infestations. This technology also purports to increase shelf life, enhance productivity, and improve nutritional value of crops.

But no long-term studies have been performed on foods produced using GMOs. Scientists are playing with and changing DNA. Essentially, cancer and other diseases are the result of something gone awry with DNA. Nobody knows whether the human body can handle this type of foreign entity made up of unnaturally created species.

With GMO crops created to withstand large amounts of herbicides and pesticides, farmers will indeed use those products to increase productivity. That means you'll consume produce (or animals fed that produce) grown with increased amounts of harmful chemicals. Risks involved with digesting some of these compounds are well documented.

Also, many people have life-threatening allergies to certain foods. If scientists cross-transfer genes, unsuspected exposure to the allergens is a huge possibility. If these biotechnologists splice a gene from a walnut into an apple, someone allergic to walnuts who eats that apple may have an allergic reaction. Experts don't know the impact of this technology yet. Strict labeling would have to be mandated to prevent potentially serious health consequences from occurring.

Nature tends to outsmart humans. With the current overuse of antibiotics (particularly in factory farming), bacteria has adapted, grown stronger, and become more resilient to these drugs. New, genetically mutated bacteria thrive and no longer succumb to the most powerful antibiotics we have. This is leading to worse infections that drugs can't keep up with. Perpetuating this logic with our food supply is like turning us all into guinea pigs in a grand experiment that puts our safety and health on the line.

As it stands now, labeling food as GMO is voluntary and not regulated by the government. Proponents of mandating labeling insist that people have the right to know what they're eating. The FDA considers GMO foods equivalent to non-GMO foods, so they are not subject to stricter labeling.

The good news for consumers is that a product *certified organic* cannot be made using GMO ingredients. But beware of products labeled "non-GMO" or "GMO-free." No laws enforce the accuracy. To avoid GMOs, purchase only organic foods.

DEFINITION

Certified organic is a labeling term that means a food or food product has been produced following the guidelines of the USDA National Organic Standards Board. Organic production is a system that integrates cultural, biological, and mechanical practices that foster cycling of resources, promote ecological balance, and conserve biodiversity.

Soy is the most common genetically modified crop used for food, followed by corn. These are also two of the most common foods used in a wide assortment of products as ingredients with various aliases.

Ingredients with soy include but are not limited to hydrolyzed vegetable protein (HVP), textured vegetable protein (TVP), textured soy protein (TSP), textured soy flour (TSF), lecithin, meat analogues, isolated soy protein, isolated vegetable protein, soy protein concentrate, and structured protein fiber (SPF). Of course, soy bran, soy fiber, soy nuts, soy oil, soy sauce, soy grits, and soy meal are also made from soybeans.

Corn-made ingredients include high-fructose corn syrup, corn syrup, corn syrup solids, malt, maltodextrin, maltose, maltol, ethyl maltol, malt syrup, mannitol, dextrose, dextrin, polydextrose, corn starch, corn flour, and corn oil.

Unless you stick with organic products, you should avoid the thousands of products made with soy- and corn-derived products. And really, until science confirms their safety, avoiding GMOs altogether is best. The potential risks involved in their consumption are simply not worth it.

Raw Resolution

Although a raw diet is nothing new, it's all the rage nowadays with raw books, products, websites, and even restaurants popping up everywhere. Defining a raw diet depends on who you ask, but a general consensus is "an eating style consisting primarily of uncooked, unprocessed foods." Some raw foodists strive to eat 100 percent of their foods raw, but technically, anything greater than 75 percent is considered a raw diet. Similarly, people who eat 50 to 74 percent of their calories from raw food sources are categorized as "high-raw foodists."

On a raw plan, foods include fresh, dried, and frozen fruits; fresh and frozen vegetables; raw nuts and seeds; and sprouted vegetables, grains, and legumes. Common preparation techniques in the raw world are soaking, sprouting, juicing, and blending. Subpopulations under the raw umbrella emphasize fruits, sprouts, and/or fermented and cultured foods.

> **MIXED GREENS**
>
> Fruitarians are a raw subgroup who eat 75 percent or more of their calories from fruit. High-fruit groups consume 50 to 74 percent of their diet from fruit. Some fruitarians eat a mono diet in which they use food-combining charts to determine which foods properly digest with others. They typically eat one to three items for their whole meal. For instance, monodieters may call 10 bananas breakfast. The goal is to optimize digestion and absorption.

Known benefits of following a raw or high-raw diet include improved nutrient intake and minimized consumption of health-damaging foods. Raw, whole foods include all the magical nutrients this book is based on: fiber, phytochemicals, antioxidants, vitamins, and minerals. Additionally, following a raw plan automatically eliminates all the harmful antinutrients: dietary cholesterol, animal protein, refined sugars, trans fatty acids, and artificial sweeteners, colors, and flavors.

Ultimately, a raw-based diet is amazing for your health. In fact, it sounds like the perfect plan. However, some concerns should be considered before you throw away your cookware.

Raw Diets Aren't Perfect

Notice that I described a raw-*based* diet—not a raw diet—as amazing in the preceding paragraph. One problem with being a strict raw foodist is that it's very difficult, and not entirely healthy, to get 100 percent of your calories from raw sources. A calorie paradox can come into play, complicating efforts to stay raw.

Fruits and vegetables are very low in calories, and you need a whole bunch of these foods to fill you up. Sprouted grains and legumes are denser in calories, but it's not as easy to eat a bowl of these raw as it is when they're cooked. Some strict raw foodists compensate for the lack of calories by consuming high amounts of fat from sources such as avocados, coconut and its oils, nuts, seeds, and other oils. High-sugar items like dried fruits and raw agave are also sometimes consumed excessively.

Raw diets lack the science to back up any of the health claims that serve as their basis. Concepts such as raw foods being live and having abundant enzymes are partially flawed arguments.

Yes, raw foods are high in plant enzymes. They are released when the plant's cell walls are broken down in chewing or blending. Enzyme activity is ripe and most lively the moment the cell walls are broken, immediately after cutting the plants with a blade or your teeth. This activity begins to slow down soon after being exposed to oxygen.

> **MIXED GREENS**
>
> Two plant enzymes—myrosinase and alliinase—help convert phytochemicals into active substances when consumed in their raw form. Myrosinase is found in cruciferous vegetables like broccoli, Brussels sprouts, bok choy, cabbage, cauliflower, and kale. Alliinase is available in allium vegetables such as onions, leeks, garlic, and chives.

But it does not appear those enzymes can survive our digestive tract long enough to have a healthy impact inside the body. The stomach, where food remains for an average of 40 minutes, is very acidic and denatures, or inactivates, enzymes before the food moves down the intestinal tract for absorption. Furthermore, whether most plant enzymes are helpful to humans is unknown, even if they did survive.

Because certain nutrients are absorbed better when cooked, exclusively raw diets cannot take advantage of these. Carotenoids such as lycopene and lutein are enhanced when heated. Cooking also breaks down some nutrients, like *oxalates*, that prevent absorption. Cooking also adds variety. Besides, eating soups, stews, and cooked grains is comforting, especially when it's cold outside.

DEFINITION

Oxalates are compounds found in plant foods, especially leafy greens, that greatly reduce the body's absorption of calcium, iron, and magnesium. Some of these oxalates can be broken down by soaking or cooking. A buildup of oxalates in the body has the potential to cause kidney stones.

Some raw foodists believe food combining is necessary for good digestion. Consuming protein and starch together is believed to be taxing on the body. It's thought that if the alkaline and acidic digestive enzymes necessary to absorb those macronutrients are expelled at the same time, they'll nullify each other, impairing digestion.

Food combining involves following a complicated chart and list of rules about which foods to eat with others. Fruits are divided into categories of sweet, acid, subacid, and melons. High-protein foods are separate from starches and nonstarchy vegetables. Originally, a set of nine rules instructed which foods to combine with others and which to eat alone.

The first problem is the fact that the stomach is always acidic and the small intestine is always alkaline. Regardless of what food you're digesting, it will always go through the same acid and then alkaline juices. Second, all whole-plant foods contain both starch and protein. Even if you eat just a banana, you're not getting pure starch, and all different types of digestive enzymes are required for digestion. Finally, no scientific evidence confirms food combining as healthier.

This isolating type of argument for food combining prohibits beneficial nutrient pairings. Vitamin C helps the body absorb iron. So eating high-vitamin-C tomatoes with spinach helps your bloodstream take in the iron. Eating a little fat along with fat-soluble vitamins is health savvy. Adding monounsaturated-fat-filled avocado to your salad filled with carotenoid-rich carrots and tomatoes enhances the absorption of the fat-soluble vitamins.

Another issue of a raw food diet may be its potentially isolating effect on your social life. It's challenging to eat out at restaurants or at friends' houses when on a raw diet.

Using Raw Sensibly

The small amount of research out on raw food diets shows mostly healthy improvements on the subjects. However, the raw food diet is a contrast against a standard disease-promoting diet. More convincing evidence would come from comparing raw diet practitioners to whole-food, plant-based eaters who include some cooked foods.

Eating a majority of your calories from raw foods is ideal. The health benefits of raw foods are indeed limitless. The idea that your diet must be *completely* raw to derive those health benefits is simply unproven.

Nutrition is regularly steeped in controversy, making food choices confusing. Misinformation is commonly—and loudly—reported by organizations that reap the benefits of their own half-truths. Be wary of dollar signs and too-good-to-be-true promises. Despite that, if you stay tuned in to reliable science and listen to your own common sense, wise eating habits are attainable.

The Least You Need to Know

- Dairy does more harm than good when it comes to your health, contributing to cancer, heart disease, and other chronic diseases.
- Calcium is abundant in plants and is bone-protective when consumed regularly along with a nutrient-dense diet.
- The soybean is a legume filled with healthy fiber and essential fatty acids.
- Eating soy from whole-food sources only and in moderation is safe.
- Following an exclusively raw diet causes some concerns, but the benefits of consuming a majority of your calories from raw foods are inarguable.

Shopping Savvy

In This Chapter

- Everything you need to know about nutrition labels
- Organic versus conventionally grown foods
- Identifying sabotaging ingredients
- Plant-based shopping

Now that you know why and how to eat whole, plant-based foods, it's time to go shopping. Filling your cart with nutritious choices is the fun part. Plus, shopping brings the theory of healthful eating to life. While at first you may feel intimidated as you carefully consider every purchase, shopping plant-based is like learning a new language. In due time, selecting the most healthful foods becomes second nature, and you'll toss items into your cart without a second thought.

In this chapter, you learn what you need to be plant-perfect (or just about). Soon you won't be able to stop talking about how great your new lifestyle is!

Reading Nutrition Labels

What I'm about to write might shock you. It goes against everything you may have heard previously. It certainly contradicts what I learned in my nutrition classes (from kindergarten through graduate school). But it will simplify your life more than any other nutrition advice ever has:

> *Never read the nutrition label on a package!*

That's right! Ignore it entirely! Everything listed there is confusing, misleading, and manipulating.

Focus on the Ingredients

The only section of a food label you should read is the list of ingredients. That's where the truth comes out. Ingredients are listed in descending order by weight (most to least). So those ingredients with the majority of the weight in the product come first, and those with the least are listed last.

Here are some tips for analyzing food products based on their ingredient lists:

- Be sure you recognize everything on the list.

- Keep it whole. Choose items with the fewest ingredients possible. The label typically shouldn't list more than three or four items. Less means more.

- Watch out for the sneaky ingredients. These include all the antinutrients, artificial anything, and items you can't pronounce.

Ultimately, most of your foods should come without ingredient lists. Vegetables and fruits are sitting out naked on the shelves in the produce section of the market; on the tables at your local farmers' market; or on the trees, bushes, and vines in your backyard. Whole grains, legumes, nuts, and seeds are sold package-free in the bulk sections or in packages with one ingredient listed.

These whole foods are the staples of your diet. Plus, shopping is faster and easier when you don't have to analyze labels!

Making Sense of Food Labels

The Nutrition Facts section on a food label intends to help you make comparisons between the nutrient contents of food products and decisions about your overall diet. The Nutrition Facts provide information on protein, cholesterol, saturated fat, dietary fiber, and other nutrients that concern your health.

The components of the nutrition panel include both mandatory and voluntary information. Disclosing numbers for calories, total fat, total carbohydrate, and sodium is mandatory. Voluntary dietary options include sugar alcohol, soluble and insoluble fiber, and other essential nutrients. The absolute amount of that nutrient found per serving in the product is listed in grams or milligrams.

Nutrition Facts
Serving Size 1 potato (148g/5.3oz)

Amount Per Serving

Calories 100   Calories from Fat 0

	% Daily Value*
Total Fat 0g	**0%**
Saturated Fat 0g	**0%**
Cholesterol 0mg	**0%**
Sodium 0mg	**0%**
Potassium 720mg	**21%**
Total Carbohydrate 26g	**9%**
Dietary Fiber 3g	**12%**
Sugars 3g	
Protein 4g	

Vitamin A 0% • Vitamin C 45%

Calcium 2% • Iron 6%

Thiamin 8% • Riboflavin 2%

Niacin 8% • Vitamin B$_6$ 10%

Folate 6% • Phosphorous 6%

Zinc 2% • Magnesium 6%

*Percent Daily Values are based on a 2,000 calorie diet.

The nutrition food label represents nutrition facts mandated by the FDA's 1990 Nutrition Labeling and Education Act.

Labeling terms like *low fat, good source of calcium, reduced sodium, lean,* and *heart-healthy* are claims defined by the FDA, and carefully determined regulations specify when foods can use these statements. The problem is that you have to look up what the terms mean in order for them to make sense. *Fat-free* doesn't mean the food is 100 percent free of fat. Instead, the FDA allows the use of the *fat-free* claim when a single serving has 0.5 grams of fat or less per serving. How much fat you consume depends on how much of the food you eat.

The same holds true for trans fats, a compound you should avoid altogether. That means a product can still legally include trans fatty acids without its label reflecting it! Most times, people eat more than one serving per meal, and therefore consume significant amounts of harmful trans fatty acids. This explains why you can see an ingredient like partially hydrogenated oil (which is, by definition, trans fat), yet the nutrition facts indicate zero trans fats. This is confusing for anyone, registered dietitians included.

The % Daily Value (%DV) column refers to how much of the specified nutrient you'll consume per serving relative to a 2,000-calorie diet. So if you're counting calories and want to be sure you're getting adequate amounts of each nutrient, you can use this column as a guideline.

One drawback of using %DV as a guideline is that not everyone eats 2,000 calories per day. Furthermore, the %DV helps only if you calculate every calorie you consume. Not only is this cumbersome and unnecessary, but how do you calculate the calories and other nutrients from, say, the salad you had at lunch? A salad usually doesn't come with a nutrition label. Technically, you'd need sophisticated nutrient software to calculate your intake accurately. And of course, you'd have to measure or weigh every portion you eat to input the correct data. No wonder diets don't work!

Nutrition Facts labels are superfluous when you eat a whole-food, plant-based diet. Your focus is quality, not quantity. You eat nutrient-dense foods when you're hungry and stop when you're satiated. Simple. No decoding, weighing, measuring, calculating, or counting necessary. Think of all that extra time you can spend being productive—finding new recipes, cooking, exercising, etc.!

Why and When to Buy Organic

The terms *organic* and *conventional* refer to the way farmers grow and process their products. Organic farming emphasizes the use of renewable and sustainable resources, with the goal of protecting the soil and water for future generations. As opposed to conventional farming, organic production abstains from using chemical pesticides, synthetic fertilizers, sewage sludge, bioengineering, or ionizing radiation.

Instead, organic farmers rely on crop rotation, biodiversity, and biological control to manage pests, maximize biological activity, and maintain long-term soil health. To be deemed certified organic, a government-approved agent must inspect and approve the farm and the protocol used in production on the farm.

Not only does this method of production protect the environment, it also benefits your body. Conventionally grown foods contain harmful pesticides such as organophosphates, which are potentially carcinogenic and toxic to the central nervous system. Organic produce also boasts higher nutrient content compared to conventionally grown foods, including protein, vitamin C, calcium, and iron.

Because of less availability and more constraints on the farmers, organic food typically costs more than conventional food. This begs the question of whether it's worth the investment.

It's definitely healthier to consume conventionally grown fruits and vegetables than not to consume them at all. Certain foods are higher in pesticides than others, so you need to prioritize what foods you buy as organic when trying to budget your purchases. For nonorganic produce, peel off the skin, if possible, and wash everything carefully with soap and water.

> **MIXED GREENS**
>
> The produce found to be highest in pesticides are known as the "dirty dozen": celery, peaches, strawberries, apples, blueberries, nectarines, bell peppers, spinach, cherries, kale, potatoes, and grapes. Buy organic of these foods whenever possible. The "clean 15" are the foods lowest in pesticides and can be purchased organic or conventionally produced. They include onions, avocados, sweet corn, pineapples, mangoes, sweet peas, asparagus, kiwi, cabbage, eggplants, cantaloupe, watermelons, grapefruits, sweet potatoes, and honeydew melons.

Organically grown produce is typically marked *organic* on the shelves. To bear the organic certification on a packaged product, food manufacturers must adhere to strict guidelines. What does an organic label on your package mean? Of course, there are other organic certifying agencies around the world, but here are the terminology and definitions required by the USDA:

- *100 percent organic* means the product is completely organic or made of all organic ingredients.

- *Organic* means at least 95 percent of the product's ingredients are organic.

- *Made with organic ingredients* means the product is made with at least 70 percent organic ingredients.

Processed products labeled "made with organic ingredients" cannot be manufactured using excluded production methods, ionizing radiation, or sewage sludge. Even when these criteria are met, the USDA organic seal may not be used on any part of the packages. Processed foods containing less than 70 percent organic ingredients may not call themselves organic on the packaging at all, but they can identify the organic ingredients on the information panel.

With such stringent regulation of organic-related labeling, it's interesting to note that the USDA doesn't standardize labeling statements such as "no drugs or growth hormones used," "free range," or "sustainably harvested." This fact is yet another justification for why you should read the ingredient list and ignore everything else.

Finding Hidden Ingredients

Ingredients you want to avoid can cleverly be hidden within food products on store shelves. They have fancy names you may not be able to pronounce, or they fall under broad categories on the label that you probably would never think of. It takes a bit of homework and a lot of practice, but soon enough, you'll be able to smell an antinutrient from an aisle away.

Products derived from animal fats and proteins are used ubiquitously, in food products, beverages, supplements, perfumes, cosmetics, skin-care products, and medications. They're even used during the production of certain products, like sugar. Because these components aren't found in the product itself, they don't have to appear in the ingredient lists. This is another reason to avoid processed foods.

In addition to animal products, harsh chemicals are sometimes used in the production of food. For example, hydrolyzed vegetable protein is made using hydrochloric acid.

Milk products are hidden in places where they really shouldn't be. Soy, almond, and rice cheeses almost always contain casein. This is strange, considering most people buy a cheese made from plant ingredients when they're avoiding dairy. Also, many brands of bread contain whey. Milk-containing products live under the following guises: whey, whey protein hydrolysate, casein, caseinate, butter, butter fat, cream, curds, custard, ghee, ammonium/calcium/magnesium/potassium/sodium caseinate, lactalbumin (phosphate), lactulose, lactose, milk protein hydrolysates, protein hydrolysates, nougat, and rennet.

MIXED GREENS

Because of the surge in people experiencing allergies, certain foods with high allergy-causing potential have been mandated to be included at the end of the ingredient lists. This helps you easily identify certain ingredients. Milk, nuts, wheat, egg, fish, shellfish, and peanuts are all required listings.

Gelatin, or gel, is a protein made by boiling skin, tendons, ligaments, and/or bones with water. Used as a thickener, gelatin can be found in fruit gelatin, pudding, candies, marshmallows, ice cream, cakes, and yogurts; it can also be found in the capsule holding together medication. In addition, gelatin can be used in the processing of wine. If the product says "vegan," you can be sure there's no gelatin in the product.

Glycerin, a by-product of soap manufacture, is normally made using animal fat. It can be found in foods and other products labeled as glycerin, glycerol, glycerides, glyceryls, glycreth-26, and polyglycol.

The terms *natural flavors* and *natural flavoring* can contain hundreds of different not-so-natural ingredients. They are defined by Title 21, Section 101, Part 22 of the Code of Federal Regulations as …

> the essential oil, oleoresin, essence or extractive, protein hydrolysate, distillate, or any product of roasting, heating or enzymolysis, which contains the flavoring constituents derived from a spice, fruit or fruit juice, vegetable or vegetable juice, edible yeast, herb, bark, bud, root, leaf or similar plant material, meat, seafood, poultry, eggs, dairy products, or fermentation products thereof, whose significant function in food is flavoring rather than nutritional.

With such a broad umbrella of "natural," you can't tell from which of the sources a natural flavor is derived. And because the word has no government-related regulation for use, food companies can use the term however they like. It's best to avoid products with "natural" ingredients.

Ultimately, the more processed the food, the more potential for hidden ingredients. Try to avoid processed foods as often as possible, relying more on whole, simple ingredients.

Plant-Based Supermarket Shopping

The secret to successful supermarket shopping is to focus on the perimeter of the store. If you picture the store where you usually shop, you'll notice produce is on the outside and processed foods are toward the center. Of course, this is an oversimplification because other foods you need are found in those center aisles, too. But the take-home message is to emphasize the fresh foods. Let's tour the market together, one aisle at a time.

To be efficient and cost-effective, write a list before you hit the store so that you know exactly what items you need. Remembering everything if you just wing it is impossible (unless you have a super memory). Before you leave, decide which recipes you're going to make in the next two or three days. Then write down all the ingredients you need to purchase to prepare those recipes specifically. On the list, include staples you may be running out of. Check your pantry and refrigerator to take inventory. Got your list? Now you're ready to hit the store!

Picking Your Produce

First stop, the produce section. Stock up on any and all fresh vegetables and fruits that look appealing and fresh or that you need for a planned recipe.

The produce department is where you should indulge and experiment. If you see a food that sparks your curiosity, take it home and try it! Most everyone settles into a food comfort zone, maintaining a stable handful of favorites. A plant-based diet is an opportunity to explore new, previously untried foods. Challenge yourself to step outside your comfort zone. Try a new vegetable every week. Pick out a different recipe. Soak and cook dried beans just to see how easy it can be. The more open your mind, the more you'll discover and broaden your knowledge base.

Plan to spend some time in the greens section, and your cart should end up bursting with green leaves. These superfoods have a shorter lifespan than some other vegetables, so be sure to pick them up at least once a week. Then you'll have them on hand for whenever you get the craving.

After the greens, find your other veggies. Good ones to keep stocked up on are bags of baby carrots, mushrooms, onions, bell peppers, broccoli, cauliflower, squash, celery, garlic, ginger, and potatoes of all varieties.

Find your fruits based on what you enjoy and what's available. Melons, berries, pears, pineapples, and oranges add color to your cart. Stock up on the seasonal options you look forward to all year, like figs, persimmons, and pumpkins in the fall and peaches, nectarines, and plums in the summer. The flavors of these special treats become a large part of the experience of the seasons.

Also visit the regulars with permanent locations in the produce section year-round, like bananas, apples, lettuce, cucumbers, and grapes. Don't forget your lemons and limes, which are hugely useful in so many recipes.

HEALTHY HINT

Farmers' markets are excellent places to frequent once a week. You can buy large amounts of the freshest produce for really good bargains. The produce is usually picked within the past 24 hours, so it's higher in nutrient content than the supermarket produce, which is driven to the store and spends time in the back before hitting the shelves. By buying at farmers' markets, you can eat produce with peak nutrition while supporting local business.

And don't forget the fresh herbs. Are you making Italian? Grab some basil, rosemary, and parsley. Mexican? Cilantro makes all the difference. It's good to have these and any other herbs you like on hand in the fridge because they can spice up any recipe.

Gettin' Spicy

In the spice aisle, pick up what you're out of. An exotic collection of spices can help you experiment in the kitchen. Plain salt and pepper is so passé!

From basics to blends, a shake of this or that can take your meal from blasé to fancy. A standard spice rack should contain any flavors you enjoy. Check out Chapter 18 for some spices regularly called for in plant-based recipes.

Bring on the Beans and Grains

While in the aisle with grains and legumes, have some fun. Notice how many different types of lentils you see. Pick a new one each time. Also grab some brown rice, brown jasmine rice, or wild rice. Have you discovered quinoa yet? Yum! Amaranth, barley, polenta, and millet are other, more exotic grains.

You can find tons of recipes for these foods if you want or need them, or you can get creative and play with these foods on your own. As you experiment with new foods, the plant-based world will explode in front of you. Nothing about plants is boring. You'll enjoy more variety here than in the old-fashioned, dreary, carnivorous realm.

> **HEALTHY HINT**
>
> Buy in bulk whenever possible to increase your options and save money. Specialty markets sell unique foods (usually culture-specific) at bargain prices and tend to have more bulk-buying options.

How many beans do you use on a regular basis? Have you noticed the vast selection in the bean section? Canned beans are fine to use if you don't have time to cook them from scratch. Try to find the salt-free options or, if you can't, drain and rinse them well before using.

Fun with Frozen Foods

The frozen-food section is filled with healthy, longer-lasting options ideal for a busy household. Frozen fruits and vegetables are usually flash-frozen, meaning they're frozen as soon as they're picked.

Frozen foods retain their nutrients and might even be a better choice than fresh sometimes in terms of convenience. Frozen veggies are already washed and chopped, making for easy additions to dishes. Frozen fruits are perfect for smoothies and save the washing and chopping phase normally required. Plus, they give a frosty, ice-cream effect when used in a green smoothie.

Miscellaneous Finds

Other items you can pick up in your supermarket include raw nuts, raw seeds (especially hempseeds, flaxseeds, and sesame seeds), dates, 100 percent pure maple syrup, corn or sprouted-grain tortillas, *plant-based milks*, sun-dried tomatoes, olives, tofu, tempeh, nutritional yeast, tamari, miso, vinegars (rice, balsamic, and apple cider), mustard, low-sodium vegetable broth, tea, coffee, cocoa powder, and raw cacao nibs.

> **DEFINITION**
>
> **Plant-based milks** are made from soy, almonds, rice, hemp, or oats and can be fortified with calcium, vitamin B_{12}, and vitamin D. Use them in the same fashion as cow's milk but without the health dangers.

With a bit of planning and some experience, shopping plant-based will become natural and simple. You'll find your rhythm and pick your preferences in time. Before you know it, you might even find yourself plant-perfect!

The Least You Need to Know

- Ignore the Nutrition Facts label, and instead focus on the ingredients. Choose products with the fewest items on the list and all ones you recognize.
- Choose organic whenever possible because organic is healthier for your body and the environment. (Plus, the difference in price grows smaller with increased demand.)

- While selecting foods with minimal ingredients is easiest, you should become acquainted with some of the names you need to avoid. Manufacturers find so many ways to sneak sketchy ingredients into food items.

- The majority of your shopping cart items should come from the perimeter of the store. Think colorful produce, whole grains, legumes, raw nuts, and raw seeds.

Plant-Perfect Fitness

In This Chapter

- Why you need exercise
- The physical and psychological benefits of exercise
- Program options for an effective workout
- Monitoring yourself for success

When it comes to managing your health, diet prevails. However, you can't be truly healthy unless regular exercise is a part of your life, too. Diet and exercise are the dynamic duo. Whole-plant foods flood your bloodstream with nutrients, and exercise distributes those nutrients into your cells. The innumerable benefits of staying fit make a consistent exercise program vital.

In this chapter, I explore the myriad health benefits for both mind and body resulting from exercise. I break down the separate components that together define fitness, and show you how to incorporate each one into your routine. Remember, fitness, like a healthful diet, is a process that includes continual assessment, monitoring, and progression. Your journey to excellent health requires that you keep moving!

Why Exercise?

With approximately 640 muscles all eager to contract and expand, your body was built to move. Your heart, of course, is also a muscle, and it needs regular exercise to maintain optimal function. Your body is more likely to rust out than to wear out, so move it or lose it!

Exercise encompasses several features that together define fitness—strength, cardiovascular endurance, muscular endurance, flexibility, and balance. You need to incorporate all these factors into a program to maximize results so you thrive in every way possible. Certain types of exercise incorporate several fitness components. Walking and jogging, for example, improve balance, cardiovascular capacity, and muscular endurance all at once. You can train these attributes separately or combine them for an individualized program of your choice.

From stable energy and decreased stress to improved sleep and cognitive function, exercise has an extraordinary ability to improve your life from every angle. And consistency is key. You'll find plenty of ways to design a perfect exercise program, but the truth is, doing anything is beneficial—as long as you do it regularly. This dedication keeps all organ systems in your body conditioned.

The Physical Benefits of Exercise

Nothing feels better than post-workout euphoria. Every cell in your body rejoices for the gift you've given it. Among a multitude of physical benefits, exercise ...

- Encourages nervous system communication.
- Boosts immune function.
- Increases insulin sensitivity.
- Develops positive bone turnover.
- Reduces stress.
- Protects the heart and blood vessels.
- Stimulates the endocrine system to release healthy hormones.

Metabolic Magic

Food provides all the energy your body needs for its daily functions, and consistent exercise improves your *metabolism*. Most of the energy—60 to 70 percent—is required for your *basal metabolic rate* (*BMR*), or all your body's major functions. About 10 percent of your total calories are used in the *thermic effect of food* (*TEF*).

Metabolism is the whole range of biochemical processes that occur in your body and are necessary to maintain life. **Basal metabolic rate** (**BMR**), a measure of the rate of metabolism, is the energy needed to sustain the metabolic activities of cells and tissues to maintain circulatory, respiratory, gastrointestinal, and renal processes. **Thermic effect of food** (**TEF**) is the increase in energy expenditure associated with the processes of digestion, absorption, and metabolism of food.

Your physical activity increases the amount of energy used. How much depends on your muscle mass, age, fat percentage, fitness level, weather, and duration and intensity of your exercise.

All these components of metabolism are made more efficient with exercise. Exercising improves digestion and absorption of nutrients, the number of calories expended during rest and activity, and the way your cells function.

Researchers agree that the benefits associated with regular exercise—including the metabolic boost—unquestionably promote health and longevity via limitless mechanisms. When exercising, you're using up calories to improve fitness and condition all the muscles in your body, especially your heart.

Exercise also supports weight management. Although what you eat plays the most important role in how much you weigh, exercise certainly helps, too. Muscle mass is more metabolically active, so the more muscle tissue you have, the more calories your body requires to sustain it. Even at rest, your muscles burn calories at a higher rate than they do fat tissue. During exercise, pumping blood to the muscles temporarily increases energy requirements. Then, for several hours after exercise, you enjoy a slight elevation in calorie burn. Working out turns you into a calorie-burning machine!

A common mistake people make is to eat a higher volume of food when on an exercise program. Total calories burned during and after a workout aren't enough to warrant eating large volumes of food. This dichotomy is why many people complain that they're unable to lose weight even though they consistently work out.

Immunity Influence

Immune function is greatly enhanced through exercise. People who exercise regularly report fewer colds and sick days than their sedentary peers. The reason is twofold. First, running parallel to our *circulatory system* is the *lymphatic system*. Because the lymphatic system doesn't include a pump (like the heart, which acts as the pump of the circulatory system), it relies on muscle contractions to move lymph fluids throughout the body. Exercise stimulates this process, which encourages the elimination of bacteria, viruses, and other immune stressors.

DEFINITION

The **circulatory system** consists of the heart, arteries, capillaries, and veins, and is responsible for transporting blood, oxygen, and nutrients to all cells in the body. The **lymphatic system** includes vessels and lymph nodes separate from the circulatory system that filter out microorganisms and other toxins before it returns fluid and protein to the blood. The lymphatic system carries white blood cells throughout the body to help fight infection.

Exercise also suppresses the release of stress hormones such as cortisol, adrenaline, norepinephrine, and epinephrine, which the endocrine system secretes when tension is induced. Constant stress makes you vulnerable to illness at all levels, from more colds to heart disease. Simply having an outlet for the stress through movement is also beneficial. It's impossible not to feel calmer after a workout.

Your sleep also improves with regular exercise. Moreover, it enables you to reach a deeper, more restful state when you do sleep, making repair and regeneration superior. Sound sleep is essential for immune system function, among everything else. There really is no substitute for a good night's rest.

Dodging Disease

Heart-healthy cardiovascular exercise (also known as "cardio") has a major influence over risk factors for heart attack and stroke. Consistently raising and sustaining your heart rate lowers your blood pressure, "bad" (LDL) cholesterol, and total cholesterol. Interestingly, exercise is one of the only effective ways known to raise your "good" (HDL) cholesterol levels. Working out is a far superior option to taking cholesterol-lowering medications—more benefit with no harmful side effects.

Cancer risk is also reduced with exercise. Colon, breast, endometrial, prostate, and lung cancer incidence can significantly decrease with a consistent fitness plan. This may be because exercise helps maintain ideal body weight, reduces excess hormones in your blood, moderates insulin and insulin-like growth factor-1 levels, boosts immunity, and suppresses inflammation. These are all cancer-promoting factors.

Once a cancer diagnosis is made, exercise can help improve outcome. Quality of life is enhanced, and fatigue is reduced. Physical activity boosts cancer survival and decreases chance of recurrence. It's never too late—and always advantageous—to kick up your activity to the next level.

Support your plant-fabulous diet with a consistent dose of exercise, and you'll maximize the benefits of both. Together they make the perfect team.

MIXED GREENS

Picture your HDL cholesterol as little Pac-Men gobbling up your LDL cholesterol. Having high levels of HDL in your cholesterol profile helps lower LDL, thereby decreasing your risk of disease. Exercise is the most powerful HDL booster. Most cholesterol-lowering medications aim to lower total cholesterol, but exercise improves the overall profile. The latter is more important in determining your risk for disease.

The Psychological Benefits of Exercise

An undeniable example of the interconnectedness of mind and body is the psychological response to exercise. Moving your body positively affects the way your mind functions. All you have to do is pay attention immediately after you finish your workout. *Endorphins* flood the brain and cause a rush of calm, clear, and comfortable feelings. Mood is stabilized, stress is reduced, and cognition is enhanced.

DEFINITION

Endorphins are neurochemicals produced in the body that act as natural painkillers.

But the bliss doesn't end right after your workout. Regular exercise has long-term benefits as well. A steady workout program can measurably minimize depression, anxiety, and stress while improving body image and self-confidence.

Energy doesn't always come easily. Typically, your energy levels hit peaks and valleys throughout the day, and you may struggle to keep yourself steadily vitalized. Exercise notoriously balances those waves and helps you maintain stamina all day long. Being filled with energy empowers you to be productive, sustain a level mood, handle stress, stay motivated, and sleep more efficiently. If everyone ate a whole-food, plant-based diet and exercised regularly, productivity would be unparalleled!

Choose Your Exercise

With plenty of exercise options, you can choose activities based on what you like. You'll never have a problem finding something you love—or at least something you can tolerate:

- If you thrive in a creative environment, dancing or weight training is perfect.

- If you prefer simplicity, walking, jogging, and swimming are excellent.

- Are you competitive? Sign up for a sport or a race, or take a class at the gym.

- Need variety? Try a new activity every day, developing a unique program to keep it interesting.

- Live by the ocean? Work out on the beach or take up kayaking, windsurfing, or surfing.

- Enjoy focusing on the mind-body connection? Yoga may be right up your alley. Or try martial arts, which challenges your mind and body while getting you in fighting shape.

If you have no idea what to do and feel intimidated, great personal trainers are eager to take your fitness to the next level, no matter what shape you're in. (Just be sure you choose a qualified individual—more on that later.) Ultimately, find something that makes you feel great, tickles your fancy, and keeps you going.

Let's take a look at some types of exercise so you can better choose the one that's right for you.

Cardiovascular Endurance

Technically, cardiovascular endurance is defined as the ability to increase *stroke volume* and maximize *cardiac output* while reducing your resting heart rate. Simply stated, it's a well-conditioned heart.

DEFINITION

Stroke volume is the amount of blood pumped from the left ventricle of the heart with one contraction. **Cardiac output** equals the total amount of blood flow from the heart during a specified period of time, or stroke volume multiplied by heart rate. Cardiac output is regulated by the amount of nutrients and oxygen the cells require, as well as the requirement to remove wastes.

One way to measure your progress with a cardio program is by your heart rate. On average, a resting heart rate, or the number of times your heart beats when you're completely inactive, is 60 to 80 beats per minute. In physically fit individuals, this rate is lowered.

Test for your resting heart rate first thing in the morning. Simply find your pulse, either by your carotid artery on the side of your throat or on your wrist. Have a stopwatch or a watch with a second hand on it ready. Use your pointer and middle fingers together to locate your pulse, not your thumb (it has a pulse of its own). Ideally, count the beats for an entire minute. You can also count the beats for 10 seconds and multiply the result by 6.

For maximum cardiovascular benefit, you need to keep your target heart rate between 60 and 90 percent of your maximum heart rate, or the greatest number of times your heart can beat in a minute. Your target heart rate is the recommended intensity level to ensure adequate stimulation of your cardiovascular system based on your age. Calculating target heart rate is a useful tool for setting and monitoring fitness goals. Here's the formula:

$$(220 - \text{your age}) \times .60 \text{ and } .90$$

The first number (× .60) gives you the low end of the range, and the second result (× .90) is the high end.

An easier method of determining whether you've reached your target heart rate during exercise is to note whether you're out of breath but not gasping for air. You should find it difficult but not impossible to talk.

When your body is working hard, as during exercise, your cardiac output increases to meet your body's demands, resulting in enhanced fitness. Exercises that improve cardiovascular endurance engage the large muscle groups for a sustained period of time, allowing the heart rate to remain elevated. Endurance exercises include walking, running, swimming, cycling, jumping, hiking, and using an elliptical trainer, step mill, or stationary bicycle.

The following table gives you approximate calorie burn of certain activities performed by a person weighing 120, 140, 160, and 180 pounds.

Calories Burned

Activity	Calories Burned per Minute			
	120 lb.	140 lb.	160 lb.	180 lb.
Aerobic dancing	7.4	8.6	9.8	11.1
Basketball	7.5	8.8	10.0	11.3
Bowling	1.2	1.4	1.6	1.9
Cycling (10 mph)	5.5	6.4	7.3	8.2
Dancing	2.9	3.3	3.7	4.2
Gardening	5.0	5.9	6.7	7.5
Golf (without cart)	4.6	5.4	6.2	7.0
Hiking	4.5	5.2	6.0	6.7
Jogging	9.3	10.8	12.4	13.9
Running	11.4	13.2	15.1	17.0
Sitting	1.2	1.3	1.5	1.7
Skating	5.9	6.9	7.9	8.8
Skiing (cross-country)	7.5	8.8	10.0	11.3
Skiing (downhill)	5.7	6.6	7.6	8.5
Swimming (moderate pace)	7.8	9.0	10.3	11.6
Tennis	6.0	6.9	7.9	8.9
Walking	6.5	7.6	8.7	9.7
Weight training	6.6	7.6	8.7	9.8

For improved endurance, work in a 30-minute (or more) session most, but preferably all, days of the week. You can break up the time into 10-minute intervals for an accumulated total of at least 30 minutes a day. Done every day, this adds up to approximately 600 to 1,200 calories of extra energy expended per week. Of course, this depends on many variables, including your age, weight, muscle mass, and intensity of exercise.

Strength Training

Muscular strength is the ability to exert force on a physical object using muscles. Muscular endurance is the capacity of the muscles to sustain a repeated force over a period of time. These two components are individually important, and each is trained differently.

To improve strength and muscular endurance, a force needs to be applied methodically on a regular basis. A strength-increasing program positively impacts muscle endurance. However, the inverse is not true. Emphasizing endurance won't necessarily enhance strength gains. To illustrate, imagine you want to build muscle and gain strength. You develop a program in which you progressively increase the weight used for your sets. Because you lift the weight during each set for a number of repetitions, you incidentally improve endurance.

Strength training, also called resistance training, requires the use of machines, dumbbells, barbells, tubing, or your own body weight to create a force your muscles can resist. Consistency is key, as muscle is hard to build but easy to lose. Programs vary depending on goals, but ideally, you should work each major muscle group at least once a week.

PLANT PITFALL

Strength training can lead to injury if you don't know what you're doing. If you've never worked with resistance, either hire a qualified personal trainer for a few sessions or watch a DVD or Internet instructional video on how to do certain exercises with proper form. The last thing you want to do is sustain an injury when you're trying to boost your health.

Here are some callisthenic exercises you can do (these require no or minimal equipment):

- Pull-ups
- Push-ups (on the wall, from your knees, full push-up, with feet elevated)
- Triceps dips
- Plank holds
- Abdominal crunches
- Calf raises
- Lunges (forward, stationary, walking)
- Pliés
- Squats

- Side planks

- Bear crawls

- Wall squats

- Single-leg balances

Typically, a strength-building workout consists of 2 to 4 sets of anywhere from 4 to 10 repetitions per exercise for each muscle group. As you get stronger, you must increase the weight to continue building strength. You may need to do two to four different exercises per muscle group, depending on your objectives. When you've reached your strength goals, you can maintain them by lifting the same weight but increasing repetitions when your sets start to feel too easy.

To build endurance, use a lighter weight for longer sets, with more repetitions per set. For example, you can perform 3 sets of 15 to 25 repetitions.

Stretching

Stretching is the most neglected component of fitness. Yet the benefits are infinite, and improvements happen fast if done regularly. *Flexibility* matters because it elongates muscles, which enables movement and protects the joints.

DEFINITION

Flexibility is a joint's ability to move freely through a full and normal range of motion. Many factors influence joint mobility, including genetics, the joint structure itself, neuromuscular coordination, and strength of the opposing muscle group.

The benefits of regular stretching include increased performance and decreased risk of injury. Training also increases blood supply and nutrients to the joints. This improves circulation, nutrient exchange, and the deceleration of degeneration of the joint tissues.

The most effective way to stretch is to hold each stretch for at least 30 seconds, breathe deeply, and relax into it. Be sure your body is warm before you begin by warming up with a cardiovascular activity to prevent injury. Stretch each major muscle group after you use it, and be consistent. Daily practice is best, and dedicating at least 10 minutes during each session optimizes results.

Functional Fitness

Currently "functional fitness" has inundated the workout scene. And justifiably so. Taking rehabilitation and injury prevention to the next level, exercises are specifically intended to enhance activities of daily living, such as walking, sitting up, preparing meals, eating, lifting, and bending. Essentially, it's fitness aimed at surviving and thriving in the real world by preparing the body to handle physical stress.

Training functionally usually entails a lot of core work to strengthen the muscles used to protect the back and maintain posture. (Your core is the group of muscles located around the trunk of your body—the abdominal muscles rectus abdominis, transverse abdominis, and external and internal obliques; the pelvic floor muscles; and the spinal stabilizer muscles.) Exercises that incorporate the entire body are used as well. The focus is on improving balance, strengthening the entire body, and elongating muscles.

Sports

Engaging in sports is a great way to stay in shape without even realizing it. If you have a competitive spirit or just enjoy the challenge, you can sign up to play sports locally or round up a group of friends and start a team. Whether basketball, softball, or soccer, opportunities abound for everyone from the former high school jock to the seasoned athlete.

Accountability to a team will ensure you show up. Plus, you'll be motivated to maintain your fitness level, knowing your performance depends on it. Huffing and puffing, unable to keep up with your teammates, will inspire you to keep heading to the gym.

HEALTHY HINT

Always be sure to warm up before you play a game or practice, and stretch during and afterward. Also strengthen the muscles you use in the sport on different days with resistance training to enhance performance and prevent injury.

Just Move It!

Regardless of your workout program, always include movement throughout your day whenever possible. Get creative in finding ways to do so. Consider these examples:

- Take the stairs instead of the escalator or elevator—even if it's five floors.
- Park far from the entrance of where you're going.

- While you're talking on the phone, stretch; do squats, lunges, pliés, or calf raises; or walk up and down stairs.

- When you're in your car stopped at a stop light, squeeze your glutes and your abdominal muscles until the light turns green.

- When doing dishes or brushing your teeth, do leg swings, calf raises, or abdominal squeezes.

- Drink a lot of water all day so you have to get up and walk to the bathroom more often.

- When scheduling a get-together with friends or a romantic date, include an activity like a hike, jog, or hot new fitness class. Wall climbing and salsa dancing are sexy and fun!

- While waiting in line, squeeze, hold, and release different muscles throughout your body. Nobody notices you making isometric contractions, but you improve blood and lymph flow.

- If you watch TV, stay active while doing so. Do calisthenics on the floor. Place a mini-trampoline, step, or other cardio equipment in front of the TV—and *use it!* Save movies or recorded TV shows you're excited to watch when you're exercising.

- On your way anywhere throughout the day, don't just walk. Instead, either run or do walking lunges to your destination.

- Sit on a large stability ball instead of a chair at your desk to engage your core muscles. (I wrote this entire book while sitting on my big, red stability ball.)

Go to the Gym or Work Out at Home?

You may be a gym rat or a gym-phobe—it all depends on your personality. Gym-goers like being around other people and taking classes. Each comes with its own benefits.

Working out at the gym means you have a convenient assortment of equipment options and classes. You'll find inspiration oozing from surrounding gym members, and you'll also have the opportunity to learn new exercises by watching others or asking a trainer. Plus, there's more variety at a gym than you're likely to get at home.

If you do exercise at the gym, be sure to plan your workout before you get there. Also, schedule your workouts according to the gym's less-hectic times so you can have your choice of equipment or space in the classroom. And always bring some water and a towel.

If you prefer to work out at home, you can still achieve a progressive and balanced workout program. Literally thousands of workout DVDs, podcasts, live streaming, and other high-tech options are available in every genre of fitness for rent or purchase. After some trial and error, you'll know which ones work for you and challenge you in a good way. Be sure to vary the workouts; don't get stuck on just one or two. Variety is the spice of your fitness life, so shake it up often.

You can purchase a wide assortment of workout equipment for your home, from the small and inexpensive to the large and costly. Dumbbells, foam rollers, exercise balls, and rubber tubing can fit easily into any-size home and are an affordable way to stay in shape. This equipment usually comes with instructional videos or manuals so you have an idea of how to use them. You can find additional resources online or at your local DVD-rental store.

On the other end of that spectrum are large pieces of equipment that may fit into your space and price range. Commercial-grade treadmills, ellipticals, and stationary bikes have come a long way in the last several years. So have other types of fitness equipment, like total body resistance machines and Pilates equipment. Ultimately, what matters most is finding something you either love or at least can commit to.

MIXED GREENS

Many personal trainers do in-home training. In fact, that's how I worked my way through graduate school. I spent 12 years going to people's homes and getting creative using tubing, their furniture, and even their kids to make fitness fun and effective. You can hire a certified personal trainer for a temporary period of time to help you set up a program or, if possible, on an ongoing basis to motivate, monitor, and help you progress.

Working out at home means you can wear whatever is most comfy (even your torn-up sweats) and not have to worry about what anyone thinks. Plus, there's the convenience factor—if you're home, you're at your gym! And unless you live with others who will also work out in your gym, equipment and space in the classroom are always available. As a bonus, you can enlist the support of your family members—or even your pets!

From home, you can always go for a walk, hike, jog, bike ride, or swim if you have access to a pool. Depending on the weather, you may prefer the outdoors anyway.

Fit Tips

The take-home message here is that you need to exercise. It will enhance your health in hundreds of ways and be well worth the effort. How you divide up your training (how much cardio versus strength workouts, for example) isn't as important as just doing something. Find what works for you and stick with it. The rewards will come instantly, and they'll only get better with consistency.

Keep these tips in mind while planning your workouts:

- Set goals for yourself that are realistic, measurable, and timely. Write them down, and re-evaluate them often.

- Incorporate all the components of fitness into your training regularly.

- Enlist the support of family, friends, or fellow gym-goers. Tell them your goals, and share your progress.

- Schedule your workout into your day and prioritize it. If possible, do it first thing in the morning, because excuses tend to build up as the day goes along.

- Keep your body guessing. The moment your workout feels easy, kick it up a notch. The only way to continue seeing results is to constantly challenge your body.

Monitoring Your Progress

Stay tuned in to your workout program. It should be a dynamic, fluid process that bears results immediately and continuously. You should always feel great afterward and see gains in endurance (you can go farther or for longer), strength (you can lift more or do more reps), flexibility (you can stretch farther), and balance (you can balance better). Keep track and be aware of your body.

Adaptation occurs quickly and often when you're doing what you're supposed to be doing in your workout program. Your exercise program should never feel easy. If it does, you won't benefit, and you'll get stuck in a plateau. Always consider adding more time, speed, weight, intensity, and/or frequency to keep your body challenged.

DEFINITION

Adaptation is your body's physiologic response to exercise. It occurs with a persistent training regimen and means your body has learned to cope with the stress you've placed on it from your current program. To avoid plateaus, change your workout frequently.

Another way to monitor your progress is to notice physical changes. You may weigh the same on the scale but fit better in your clothes. This is a great marker of muscle growth. Measuring yourself—chest, arm, waist, hips, thigh, and calf—affirms that your weight has redistributed. You may also be able to witness actual growth of muscles by looking in the mirror. Be sure to take note of how you feel, too.

And ask yourself some questions as you progress. Have you reached your current goals? What do you need to achieve the next goal? Assessment is crucial. Figure out what works and what doesn't. Problem-solve until you figure out what works best for you to attain your goals.

To achieve optimal health, you need a clean diet, plenty of rest, and relaxation or stress-management skills. Exercise completes the equation and adds quality to your life, pep to your step, and clarity to your mind. Embrace regular exercise—if you haven't already—and you will thrive.

The Least You Need to Know

- Incorporating exercise into your days boosts the benefits of a plant-based diet.
- Being fit incorporates cardiovascular and muscular endurance, strength, flexibility, and balance. Include exercises to improve all these.
- It doesn't matter where or what you prefer—find any exercise program you love and will stick to, and then commit to it.
- Keep your body on its toes. As soon as something becomes easy, change it up so you continue to challenge yourself and reap the benefits.

To Supplement or Not to Supplement?

In This Chapter

- Micronutrients to consider
- Getting your vitamin B_{12} and D
- Current research on supplements
- The brilliance of your body

The most commonly asked question in nutrition today is whether or not supplements are necessary. In this multibillion-dollar industry, supplement manufacturers have confused the public beyond comprehension. You probably worry about whether you're getting enough nutrients from your diet alone—especially on a plant-based plan. How do you know if you're getting enough of each nutrient? Who can you trust for unbiased information? If you need a supplement, which type do you choose? Is taking more better than not taking enough? Are they safe?

In this chapter, we examine these questions in detail.

Do You *Need* to Supplement?

Everyone is unique in genetic makeup, habits, daily food intake, and health choices. So it's impossible to say that nobody or everybody needs to supplement. Many factors determine whether your diet meets your nutrient needs.

Supplements need to be considered and treated as medications. If you have a nutrient deficiency, you need to determine what the origin of that deficiency is. Most of the time, a nutrient deficiency signifies either a health issue or a poor diet overall. In either of these cases, popping a supplement won't address the real problem.

Additionally, nothing comes without risk. Every drug has associated side effects, and most of the science available shows that supplements don't make you healthier. That being said, a whole-food, plant-based diet that contains a wide variety of different foods every day should provide everything you need, with the exception of vitamin B_{12} and possibly vitamin D.

Boosting Your B_{12}

Vitamin B_{12} deficiency in herbivores is rare but serious. No gold standard exists to test for blood cobalamin deficiency. Currently, the most commonly used tests are MMA (methylmalonic acid) and homocysteine. Ask your physician to test you during your regularly scheduled visits.

If you're plant based, be sure you're taking a B_{12} supplement of at least 5 to 10 micrograms per day. Or be adamant about regularly consuming fortified products such as nutritional yeast or plant milks to ensure adequate intake. Although the RDA for B_{12} is only 2.4 micrograms, supplements are not completely absorbed; this is why the recommendation for intake is higher.

Two different types of B_{12} compounds are available as supplements: methylcobalamin and cyanocobalamin. Although most commercial products use cyanocobalamin, when choosing a vitamin B_{12} supplement, seek out the methylcobalamin version. Methylcobalamin is better absorbed, is retained in your body's tissues longer, and doesn't leave a poisonous cyanide molecule to deal with after it's metabolized in the body like cyanocobalamin. Chewing vitamin B_{12} tablets improves absorption, but the under-the-tongue versions are absorbed well, too. You can also ask your doctor for an injectable B_{12} if you have any absorption issues.

Do's and Don'ts of Vitamin D

Vitamin D is not as cut and dried as vitamin B_{12}. A vast majority of the world's population has either insufficient or deficient levels of vitamin D. But this doesn't mean you should just pop a pill. Before you do anything, have your 25-hydroxyvitamin D blood level tested. If you end up with a result lower than 35 to 50 ng/mL, you need to figure out how best to bring it up. Try using the sun as your first line of defense.

Everyone responds differently to sun therapy, depending on factors such as latitude where you live, skin color (the lighter your skin, the easier you will absorb vitamin D), time of year, and weather. If you live somewhere that gets a lot of sunshine throughout the year, you're at an advantage and might not have to supplement.

To maximize sun exposure safely …

- Go out during the peak time of the day, when the UVB rays are strongest, usually between 10 A.M. and 2 P.M.

- Protect your eyes with sunglasses.

- Apply sunscreen to your face to prevent wrinkling, but do not wear it on the other exposed parts of your body.

- Expose as much of your skin as possible without offending your neighbors.

- Never allow your skin to burn or even turn pink. The darker your skin, the more sun exposure you require to make vitamin D, and the harder it is for you to burn.

- Do this two or three times a week at minimum.

After following these suggestions for a couple months, take a follow-up blood test. If your results go up, congratulations! Continue with the sun exposure regimen. However, if you're unable to raise your 25-hydroxyvitamin D to at least 35 ng/mL, continue with the sun exposure, but add a vitamin D supplement.

Note this trial works best during the warmer months and in warmer climates. If you're performing the sun exposure trial during the heart of winter, you probably won't increase your levels. Your result may be situation-based and not a reflection of your personal ability to make vitamin D. Test this during the spring or summer seasons for optimal results. You might need to supplement only in the colder months.

Vitamin D_2 is a vegan source made from yeast, while vitamin D_3 is derived from animals. Conflicting information brings into question whether D_2 is as absorbable as D_3, but the consensus is that the two forms are equally effective at raising blood levels. The only caveat is that you may need higher doses of vitamin D_2 to achieve the same results you would with D_3. You can safely take 5,000 to 6,000 IU per day for two to three months. After that, level out to a maintenance dose of 1,000 to 2,000 IU per day.

PLANT PITFALL

Never double up on a multivitamin to attain optimal levels of vitamins B_{12} or D. You'll be doubling up on other compounds, too, which can be toxic.

Besides vitamins B$_{12}$ and D, you generally don't need to worry about any other supplements. It's optimal to have your blood tested for potential deficiencies common in the general population, including DHA, iron, zinc, and iodine. But as a universal rule, don't supplement "just in case." Instead, get your nutrients from your food and monitor your blood levels regularly to confirm your nutrient intake is sufficient.

The Dangers of Supplementation

In addition to cashing in on nutrient fears, supplement manufacturers imply their products can perform miracles for your health. Herbs, botanicals, blends, powders, bars, and potions promise to stop aging, prevent cancer, replace exercise, and make you popular. If it sounds too good to be true, it most definitely is.

The Dietary Supplement Health and Education Act

A major force influencing the supplement industry is a piece of legislation called the Dietary Supplement Health and Education Act (DSHEA). Passed in 1994, this act took away responsibility from the government to ensure the safety of a product before it's put on the market. Instead of the FDA determining safety, as it does for foods and medications, the drug manufacturer is in charge of its own products.

If a problem comes up after a product makes it onto the shelves, only then does the FDA become responsible. But until then, buyer beware! The only person who decides whether a supplement is safe is the same person who benefits from you buying and using it. This possible conflict of interest has broad implications.

What's Up in Supplements?

Unless you have a deficiency, supplements don't make you healthier. In certain cases, the opposite is true. Beta-carotene, vitamin E, and folic acid have been found to be harmful in numerous trials.

After the discovery that people who ate more fruits and vegetables developed less cancer, researchers were on a mission to find out precisely what component in those foods caused the prevention. This made antioxidants all the rage in the nutrition world. In the mid-1990s, two well-designed studies compared a group at high risk for lung cancer (smokers and those exposed to asbestos) taking beta-carotene and vitamin A supplements with a control group taking no supplements. Much to the dismay of the researchers, the groups taking the supplements started developing lung cancer and dying more than the control group. They had to stop the study prematurely.

Several explanations are possible, but the results are still not completely understood. Perhaps it was due to the lack of synergistic compounds found in food sources of vitamin A. Or maybe it was because out of approximately 563 identified carotenoids, taking a large dose of only one of them (beta-carotene) prevented the others from working. The lesson to be emphasized is that isolating and concentrating a nutrient doesn't have the same effect as eating it in its original packaging.

Taking large amounts of vitamin E to ward off Alzheimer's disease and prevent oxidation is popular. But in a large meta-analysis of 19 studies performed in 2005, vitamin E was found to "increase all-cause mortality" at high doses "and should be avoided." Not only do you risk dying by taking these supplements, but many studies have shown that they don't even work to begin with.

Obstetricians advise their pregnant patients to take 400 micrograms of folic acid every day to help prevent neural-tube defects in their babies. Unfortunately, research shows that taking supplemental folic acid increases the risk of breast cancer. It may also lead to a higher risk of dying from breast cancer, as well as from all causes.

It's not the nutrient itself causing these results. Instead, it's the fact you're taking it in an unnaturally isolated, concentrated form. When consumed in its original packaging—surrounded by fiber and other nutrients—the *synergy* among all the compounds working together creates magic in your body.

DEFINITION

Synergy is the effect of two or more units working together to produce a result not obtainable by each of the units independently.

Currently, taking fish oil supplements to attain high levels of the essential fatty acid DHA is the trend. Fish are the most polluted organisms. Their muscles and livers are filled with PCBs, dioxin, mercury, organochlorines, pesticides, and DDT. All these compounds provide serious health risks to humans. If you think about it, eating one fish for dinner provides you with a dose of these toxins. In the food chain, bigger fish eat smaller fish, and those bigger fish absorb the toxins from the smaller fish. Now if you concentrate the oil from hundreds or thousands of big fish and put it into a capsule, consuming that capsule concentrates your exposure exponentially!

Lawsuits have been filed over fish oil supplement manufacturers providing these toxins in their products. Even with the highly regarded molecular distillation process, products have still been found to contain these detrimental compounds. So far, not enough research has been done to confirm the potential health risks from taking these supplements.

Why chance it, especially when you don't need to take fish oil supplements in the first place? Most people can achieve optimum DHA levels by consuming plant sources of ALA (flaxseeds, hempseeds, chia seeds, walnuts, and soybeans). If after diligently eating ALA-rich foods your blood test still shows you're deficient, consider taking available microalgae formulas, a safer option than fish oil.

Knowing When to Supplement and When to Eat

The human body is the most unmistakable example of synergy. It contains trillions of cells, all communicating with one another all the time. The complexity of our bodies leaves even the most knowledgeable experts in awe. So many mysteries lie unsolved that we're only just beginning to scratch the surface of how exactly the body functions.

When consumed, the thousands of phytochemicals a plant contains become a part of your trillions of cells through complex, interrelated mechanisms. How, then, can you expect one isolated, concentrated compound—a vitamin, for instance—to cure disease? Yet that's precisely what the supplement industry claims. This ignores the intricate, complicated, and synergistic workings of the human body.

We are sick and overweight because of the way we eat, not because of micronutrient deficiency. You're more likely to see someone with heart disease than scurvy (vitamin C deficiency), cancer than beriberi (thiamin deficiency), and diabetes than pellagra (niacin deficiency). Popping supplements will never replace the effectiveness of eating whole-plant foods and exercising regularly for achieving and maintaining optimum health. You can't counteract a poor diet by taking pills. Unfortunately, it just doesn't work.

Returning to the best health quote of all time, Hippocrates' "Let thy food be thy medicine, and thy medicine be thy food" says it all. Whole-plant foods are vessels for optimum health. As humans, we're designed to take our sustenance from the planet we live on, not to create supernutrients in order to thrive.

Nor are our bodies capable of taking in massive amounts of a single substance, which is essentially what happens when we supplement. The high concentration of nutrients in supplements overloads the body. Breaking down and absorbing this vast amount is simply too much for your body to handle. One of two things happens: the extra is excreted in your urine, which is altogether wasteful, or it accumulates in your storage organs (kidneys, liver, fat), where it can ultimately reach toxic levels.

The perfection of nature is shown in infinite ways: the growth pattern of a leaf, the colors of a rainbow, cloud formations, the birth of a baby, and the brilliant mechanisms behind how your body functions. The harmony between the earth and your body is inarguable. When you eat straight from nature, it's no coincidence that you thrive. Instead of spending so much time and money trying to outsmart this harmony, embrace it and simply eat whole-plant foods.

The Least You Need to Know

- Your individual nutrient needs are based on genetics, age, makeup of your diet, and other factors.
- Vitamin B$_{12}$ is the only nutrient not available on an herbivore diet. Take it to prevent deficiency.
- Get your 25-hydroxyvitamin D blood level checked regularly, and treat deficiency with sun first and perhaps supplements additionally.
- The DSHEA Act of 1994 gave dietary supplement manufacturers, not the FDA, the power to determine their own products' safety.
- Ample research shows dangerous effects of taking supplemental beta-carotene, vitamin E, and folic acid.

Special Considerations

At all stages of life, from the womb to the senior years, nutritional requirements for your body adjust in subtle ways. During pregnancy, you need more of certain vitamins, minerals, and overall calories. In the later decades, you might need more vitamins and minerals but fewer calories. Then there are all the years in the middle. Between picky toddlerhood and stubborn adulthood, consider whole-plant foods your best ally. You literally are what you eat, so if you optimize every decade by eating the right foods, you'll thrive!

Beyond the timeline, Part 3 identifies the nutrient needs of other unique considerations. From athletes, who epitomize the pinnacle of what the human body can achieve, to people fighting disease, I offer suggestions on what does your body best.

I also provide a chapter about weight loss so you can better understand the current worldwide epidemic of obesity and overweight, which impacts every population—and maybe you. No matter your age or state of health, food matters.

Plant-Based Pregnancy and Beyond

In This Chapter

- Plant-based and pregnant!
- What to eat, how much weight to gain, and how to modify your workout
- The benefits of breast milk
- Do's and don'ts of starting on solids

Congratulations on being pregnant! Whether or not this is your first pregnancy, get set for that journey into the unknown—the exciting roller-coaster ride that comes along with making another human being. You never know what to expect as your body undergoes major, miraculous changes. All you can do is ride the waves and provide your body and the body of your growing baby with excellent nutritional support.

In this chapter, I explain precisely what a plant-based mama needs to support a developing baby. Throughout pregnancy, your body changes, and so do your needs. Knowing which substances to avoid, which foods provide the right nutrients, and how to safely continue exercising are all laid out for you here. This chapter also takes you from conception through the first year, describing how you can best set up your baby's health for life.

Growing a Healthy Baby

Your baby's health is predetermined months—if not years—before conception. Both what you eat and what you avoid directly impact the future well-being of your baby. A whole-food, plant-based diet during gestation and throughout the first 10 years is the gift that continues to give for the entirety of your child's life.

So many things have to go right to create a healthy baby. Your little human starts from the union of two cells, dividing and transforming over a series of millions of processes during the course of 9 months—or, more accurately, 40 weeks. Aside from the nausea, heartburn, constipation, discomfort, and weight gain, you're largely unaware of all the events taking place inside your womb. What can you do to help your body have everything it needs for the ultimate creation?

First, you should avoid the following, which are harmful to the developing fetus:

Caffeine: Limit your total caffeine intake from tea, coffee, soda, and chocolate to no more than 200 milligrams per day. Be careful of herbal teas because many contain medicinal effects. Mint and ginger teas, however, are safe and may help ease some of the digestive woes brought about during pregnancy.

All alcohol: No amount of alcohol consumed during pregnancy is considered safe.

Nicotine: Cigarette smoke from direct or indirect sources is dangerous.

Medications, herbs, and supplements (especially vitamin A): Be sure to tell your obstetrician (OB) about every medication, herb, and supplement you're on before pregnancy. Even over-the-counter medications, like painkillers, anti-inflammatories, and cough suppressants, can be harmful to your fetus. Discuss this in detail with your physician.

Artificial sweeteners: Use of any artificial sweeteners during pregnancy has not been proven safe.

Nitrites and nitrates: These cancer-causing compounds are found in processed (faux) meats, hot dogs, and bacon. Read the ingredient lists.

Fish, raw dairy, raw eggs, and soft cheeses: If you're on a whole-food, plant-based diet, you're already avoiding these.

Nonfood items to avoid include radiation, hot tubs, saunas, cat litter, household cleaners, paint, and any other chemicals.

In addition, take these actions to support your body during pregnancy:

- Gain the right amount of weight—no more and no less.

- Be mindful and prudent regarding your nutrient intake.

- Continue your prepregnancy exercise program, but with appropriate modifications.

- Get plenty of rest.

Pregnancy is a very special time in your life, when taking proper care of yourself is more crucial than ever. Prioritize your health, and both you and your baby will reap the benefits.

Gaining Weight Wisely

The extra calories needed during pregnancy go toward creating new tissue in the fetus, placenta, uterus, and breasts, and also to make amniotic fluid and blood. But contrary to popular belief, your calorie needs aren't greatly increased during pregnancy.

Gaining the right amount of weight creates an ideal condition for both you and your baby. Not gaining enough can lead to poor growth or nutrient deficiencies for your baby. On the other hand, gaining too much weight puts you at risk for *gestational diabetes (GDM)*, more discomfort during pregnancy, and a difficult time losing the extra weight after delivery.

> **DEFINITION**
>
> **Gestational diabetes (GDM)** is any degree of glucose intolerance that's first discovered during pregnancy. Although the condition usually resolves after delivery, it increases your long-term risk of developing type 2 diabetes. Children of moms with GDM are at increased risk of obesity, glucose intolerance, and diabetes in late adolescence and young adulthood. GDM complicates approximately 7 percent of pregnancies, according to the American Diabetes Association.

Calorie needs increase throughout the trimesters. During your first trimester, you don't need to increase calories. This is the time to find ways of consuming adequate amounts of the vital nutrients despite nausea and fatigue. When your second trimester begins, increase your intake by approximately 340 calories per day. During this period, you should be adjusting to pregnancy. Typically, nausea and fatigue subside before any discomfort from weight gain begins, allowing you to eat more nutrient-dense meals. Use the slightly elevated caloric needs to take in more vegetables and fruits. When you reach your third trimester, your baby's weight gain occurs more rapidly. Add about 452 more calories a day to your diet to support his or her growth.

As you can see, the numbers aren't that large. One cup of brown rice with a cup of steamed broccoli and an apple makes up 340 calories. Of course, when you're pregnant with more than one baby, your calorie needs are slightly higher. Ideally, you'll only gain 2 to 4 pounds during the first trimester and then between 1 and 1½ pounds per week for the remaining time. Ultimately, how much weight you should gain depends on your prepregnancy weight, your age, and the number of babies you're carrying.

The following guidelines support the health of both mother and baby.

Pregnancy Weight Gain Recommendations

Body Type	Weight (lb.)
Normal weight	25 to 35
Underweight (< 90 percent ideal body weight)	28 to 40
Overweight (> 90 percent ideal body weight)	15 to 25
Obese (> 135 percent ideal body weight)	15
Adolescent	30 to 45
Normal weight, carrying twins	35 to 45

If you're carrying multiples (more than two) during your pregnancy, weight gain recommendations may change. Your OB will provide you with some suggestions. Regardless of how many babies you're carrying, remember that these numbers are merely guidelines. Allow your body to be your guide. When you're hungry eat, but be careful not to overeat. Your focus should be on taking in the most nutrient-dense foods to meet your needs throughout your pregnancy.

Necessary Nutrients During Pregnancy

Unlike calories and weight gain recommendations, nutrient demands amplify greatly during pregnancy. Your body takes some nutrients directly out of its own storage; others you need to consume regularly from your diet. To prevent deficiency in both yourself and your baby, be sure to emphasize the following nutrients:

- Protein
- DHA
- Iron
- Vitamins A, C, B_6, and B_{12}
- Folate
- Niacin
- Riboflavin
- Thiamin
- Iodine
- Iron
- Zinc
- Selenium

Protein needs increase during the second and third trimesters to support tissue and fluid production. You need to consume approximately 25 grams more protein per day at this time (50 grams if you're carrying twins). Nutrient-rich sources include beans, leafy greens, nuts, and seeds.

Omega-3 fatty acids are critical for fetal brain development. The fetus takes in approximately 50 to 60 milligrams (mostly from DHA) during the last trimester. Maintain your stores of DHA by consuming walnuts, flaxseeds, hempseeds, chia seeds, and whole soy foods daily.

MIXED GREENS

In Chinese medicine, daily intake of walnuts is recommended during pregnancy because a walnut looks like the brain. Coincidentally, walnuts are filled with alpha-linolenic acid—the type that converts to the brain-building DHA.

Many women become iron-deficient for the first time during pregnancy. Iron needs at this time are nearly double what they are normally: you require 27 milligrams per day during pregnancy, as opposed to the usual 15 milligrams. All the extra blood essential for you and your baby increases your need to build hemoglobin. Emphasize iron-rich foods like your go-to leafy greens, making sure to eat them with a vitamin C–rich source, like tomatoes or citrus fruit.

However, achieving the RDA might not always be possible; supplementing might be necessary temporarily. Iron-deficiency anemia in pregnancy can lead to premature deliveries and low-birth-weight infants. Deficiency almost always resolves after delivery, especially because women typically have several months without having a menstrual cycle postpregnancy. This allows the body time to restore iron levels to normal.

If you must take a supplement based on your obstetrician's recommendations, drink plenty of water and eat extra fiber to compensate for the constipating effects of concentrated iron. Also, take the iron supplements between meals and separate from tea, coffee, calcium supplements, fortified foods, and legumes.

Folic acid supplements, or prenatal vitamins containing folic acid, are given to women preventively if they're even thinking about becoming pregnant. Adequate amounts of folic acid are essential in the first few weeks of pregnancy to prevent neural tube defects, typically a time before a woman discovers she's pregnant.

In Chapter 10, I explain how folic acid supplements are harmful. However, if you're adamant about consuming your greens and beans every day, you'll never have to worry about having enough folate. A cup each of raw greens, cooked greens, and lentils eaten in a day provide more than enough folate to meet your daily requirement. You can easily reach your daily folate need of 400 micrograms when you enjoy the plant sources of folate shown in the following table.

Folate

Food	Folate (mcg)
Lentils, 1 cup cooked	358
Pinto beans, 1 cup cooked	294
Spinach, frozen, 1 cup cooked	230
Turnip greens, raw, 1 cup	107
Orange juice, raw, 1 cup	74
Collard greens, raw, 1 cup	60
Broccoli, raw, 1 cup	50

To maintain all your nutrient levels throughout your pregnancy, stay on top of your usual whole-food, plant-based plan. Be sure you're taking your vitamin B_{12} via supplement or fortified sources, and be sure your vitamin D levels are up to par. Part of routine prenatal care includes testing for micronutrient deficiency (especially iron). If you were deficient before pregnancy, odds are, you'll stay deficient, and may even become worse, during pregnancy. It takes a village of nutrients to create a little human. Be sure your village is well stocked.

Exercise During Pregnancy

Your body changes in more ways than you can predict during a pregnancy, regardless of how many times you've been through it. Structural changes occur to allow the baby to grow, expand, and, ultimately, come out to meet you. Hormones are released to enable these changes, helping relax your joints, mobilize your bones, and generally open up. The more in tune you are with your body going into pregnancy, the more control you can exert over how you handle these changes.

Being fit from the get-go is a huge advantage. You're able to continue exercising, reaping the multitude of benefits that come from maintaining your fitness level throughout pregnancy, including the following:

- Improved circulation

- Weight management before and after pregnancy

- Energy maintenance

- Better sleep quality

- Minimized joint discomfort from weight gain

- Ability to maintain endurance, strength, and flexibility

- Easier delivery

- Improved recovery postdelivery

Still, you must tailor how you work out to your pregnancy. During the first trimester, you can pretty much maintain what you were doing prepregnancy. Of course, at this time, most women are bogged down by major fatigue and nausea, thanks to the dramatic hormonal shifts. So listen to your body, and of course, speak with your OB about what you're currently doing. Move your body as much as is comfortably possible.

PLANT PITFALL

Pregnancy is not the time to work on strengthening your abdominal (stomach) muscles. Not only does it put strain on your womb, but you don't want those muscles to be shortened and tight. Your abdominal cavity needs to expand at this time to allow room for the baby. Instead, focus your strengthening efforts on your back, arms, and legs. You'll have plenty of time to regain your ab muscles postdelivery, once you get the go-ahead from your OB.

During the second trimester, you should begin to ease out of the fatigue and nausea before you experience the discomfort of carrying around extra weight—in a very awkward place on your body with respect to gravity. This is the perfect time to move more. Walking and using an elliptical, stationary bicycle, or step mill are great ways to get in your cardio. Running is not ideal because jumping may be jarring on your baby and your own body. Running also puts you at higher risk of falling because your center of gravity has shifted.

Lifting light to moderate weights is excellent to maintain muscle mass. Just be extremely careful with your form. It's easier to sustain an injury because your joints are abnormally relaxed. Don't try to lift heavier weights than you did before pregnancy; it may be best to do lighter-weight, higher-rep workouts. Hit all your major muscle groups at least a couple times a week.

Stretching should feel fabulous at this point. You may be able to stretch farther than ever before in your life—even as a child! Just be gentle, and don't force anything. But working on your flexibility (especially in your hips) may help with delivery.

It's important to remember during exercise that after 20 weeks, you should refrain from lying on your back because this can interfere with blood flow to your baby and placenta. Plenty of exercises can be performed in an incline position. Use a workout bench or firm pillow to raise your head, shoulders, and back to a good angle that will protect your baby and enable you to hit muscle groups like your chest.

During your final trimester, everything changes. This is the time when your weight gain is the greatest. You may slow down and feel achy or uncomfortable. If you can, continue some form of movement. Swimming is perfect because it provides that feeling of weightlessness and gives you an opportunity for relief while getting your heart rate up.

Everyone is unique, and that affects many variables during pregnancy. I will never forget a woman who, at 9 months pregnant, was doing headstands in my yoga class. On the other extreme, those who gain a lot of weight can barely waddle through their day. Multiple pregnancies (twins or more) add extra stress to the body and should be monitored closely.

Your goal during the last few weeks is to stay comfortable, maintain movement as much as possible, and listen to your doctor's orders. Preterm labor can have potential health implications for your baby, so you want to be sure he or she is fully cooked before it's time to come out. Intense exercise has the potential to increase contractions, and you don't want to push yourself into early labor just to keep up with your routine.

PLANT PITFALL

If exercising brings on contractions, pain, or bleeding, stop your activity and call your OB immediately.

Walking usually feels good and improves circulation to you and your baby. Lifting light weights also enhances blood flow and helps maintain strength and functionality. Gentle stretching may help open your joints and relieve tension. During this time, be sure to get plenty of rest. Take special care of your body, and listen to its signals closely. Before you know it, you'll be holding your little one, finally having that opportunity to see who has been growing inside of you.

Postpregnancy is a great time to ease your way back into your old routine after your OB grants approval. Remember that your body has undergone major construction and deconstruction, and it may take a while to get your stamina back. Your fitness level postpregnancy depends on how fit you were beforehand. Take it one workout at a time, and your endurance, strength, and flexibility will return to normal along with your weight. Remember that it took 9 months to gain the weight, and it takes about the same amount of time, on average, to take it off. Stay consistent, and you'll see results.

Tips to Nip Nausea and Other Discomforts

The power of hormones becomes ragingly obvious the moment you become pregnant. Initially, your body surges with estrogen, progesterone, and human chorianic gonadotropin (HCG)—hormones that help maintain the pregnancy. This hormonal influx causes the feeling of nausea and sometimes vomiting. Some strategies help alleviate these symptoms.

Nausea is greater when your stomach is empty. This explains why it's typically called "morning sickness," although the nausea can, and usually does, occur throughout the day. You wake up with no food in your stomach after an overnight fast. Eating small, regular meals throughout the day helps moderate this feeling. To help break the fast, you can keep crackers by your bedside to eat the moment you wake up.

You may notice that bland, starchy, and salty foods are the easiest to tolerate. A risky consequence of nausea is the inability to consume a wide variety of nutrient-dense foods. Do the best you can. Take advantage of less-nauseous times of the day to eat as many micronutrient-rich foods as you can find (greens, beans, veggies, and fruits).

Also, keep the following in mind:

- Soups may be easier to tolerate than raw veggies.
- Whole-grain crackers provide more nutrients than white crackers.
- To stave off nausea, sip ginger tea or chew on ginger candy.

- Try sipping carbonated water.

- Continue drinking liquids to prevent dehydration, especially if you're vomiting.

- See your OB if you're unable to keep down any food or liquids.

> **HEALTHY HINT**
>
> Ginger root is one of the very few herbs considered safe during pregnancy. It's helpful in alleviating nausea. Boil fresh ginger root in hot water for a delicious tea, buy 100 percent ginger tea bags at the store, or chew on ginger candies when you feel nauseous.

Another source of discomfort that comes with pregnancy is heartburn. Heartburn is the symptom that coincides with stomach acid being released into the esophagus. Pregnancy-induced spikes in progesterone relax the esophageal sphincter, and the uterus puts pressure on the stomach. To help ease the discomfort, follow these tips:

- Eat your meals slowly.

- Avoid getting too full by eating small, frequent meals throughout the day.

- Stay upright for at least a couple hours after you eat so the food has time to pass through your upper GI tract.

- Avoid acidic foods or those high in fats.

Constipation is another very common occurrence during pregnancy. A number of factors can contribute to the issue. It's partly those darn hormones again. Progesterone decreases muscle contractions, which slows down the movement in the intestines. A growing fetus takes up space and can interfere with normal bowel movements, too. If you're taking iron supplements, you have yet another variable keeping you stopped up.

Be sure you eat lots of fiber (impossible not to do on a whole-food, plant-based diet) and drink plenty of water. Exercise also helps.

Plantlings: Raising Healthy Babies

Congratulations! After those long, intense, challenging, and sometimes uncomfortable 40 weeks, you finally get to meet and hold your baby. As you gaze into his or her eyes, you may be thinking, *So now what?*

You have the power to provide your baby with one of the greatest gifts a mother could ever give her child—superior nutrition for lifelong health! Diet in the first decade of a child's life is more significant than all the remaining years of his or her life. Massive growth occurs during these years, and cells divide at a rapid pace. This is a period of great opportunity to provide your child's cells with optimal nourishment. And a nutrient-dense diet lays the groundwork for powerful immunity and a healthy future.

Breast Milk or Formula?

The very first decision you make after your baby is born (if you didn't decide before the birth) is whether you plan to breastfeed. Nothing is healthier for an infant than mother's milk. It's tailor-made for just your baby, complete with your immune system and nutrients from your plant-based diet. With a world of unique benefits, your breast milk …

- Provides antibodies that form the basis of your baby's immune system.

- Supports brain development with optimal nutrient levels (including DHA).

- Encourages good, health-promoting bacteria to form in your baby's intestinal tract.

- Offers *passive immunity* to protect your baby from infections until he or she develops his or her own immune system.

DEFINITION

Passive immunity is temporary protection against disease gained when one human gives already-made antibodies to another via breast milk.

- Sustains long-term health advantages, such as preventing allergies, ear infections, both types of diabetes, multiple sclerosis, childhood cancers, Crohn's disease, overweight/obesity, and many other health problems.

- Gives a cost-effective alternative to formula—it's free!

- Is convenient—always ready to eat!

- Promotes easier postpartum weight loss for you.

- Decreases your risk of premenopausal breast cancer.

The most critical moment of breastfeeding is immediately after your milk comes in. Colostrum, the first milk to be secreted after your baby is born, is liquid gold. It's rich in antibodies that coat your baby's intestinal tract, setting up the immunity foundation.

The American Academy of Pediatrics (AAP) recommends breast milk as the sole source of food for the baby's first 6 months and then a combination of breast milk and supplemental foods for the rest of the first year. Some experts recommend breast-feeding through the age of 2, although all the health benefits have been bestowed after 1 year. Ultimately, the more breast milk you offer your baby, the better. Continue for as long as you can up until the age of 2.

Some women are unable to breastfeed due to physical or other obstacles. If this is the case, available plant-based infant formulas are fortified with all necessary nutrients. Be certain to choose one with added DHA.

Nutrify Your Breast Milk

Your breast milk is a direct reflection of what you eat. Nutrient content and toxin concentration change based on food consumption. This puts you in the driver's seat; you can maximize nutrition in your baby the entire time you breastfeed. Breast milk from strict plant-eaters is adequate in nutrients as long as you're actively taking a vitamin B_{12} supplement.

HEALTHY HINT

If you're not supplementing with 5 to 10 micrograms vitamin B_{12} while breast-feeding, give your baby liquid B_{12}: 0.4 micrograms per kilogram body weight every day.

To boost the nutrition level of your breast milk, eat a wide variety of plants. Also avoid all chemicals in your food, drinks, and everyday life. Remember, if you wouldn't give it directly to your baby, don't expose yourself to it either. Stick to the goal of eating high on the nutrient-density continuum by basing your meals on greens, beans, other vegetables, fruits, whole grains, nuts, and seeds. Consume at least two sources of omega-3 fatty acids—walnuts, hempseeds, flaxseeds, chia seeds, and whole soy products—every day.

Not only are you kick-starting your baby's health, but you're also introducing tastes to your baby's pure palate. Odds are, if you love your greens and eat them daily during breastfeeding, your baby will, too. What a great way to start life!

The First Year: Nutrition No-No's

During the first year or two of life, certain foods should be avoided. No type of milk other than breast milk or baby formula is safe for your baby until after 1 year of age. This includes all types of dairy and plant-based milks.

Allergies and colic can show up in the form of gastrointestinal symptoms, rashes, or persistent crying. If you, the baby's father, or his or her siblings have a history of severe food allergies, monitor your baby carefully while breastfeeding and note any new foods eaten recently that may have caused a reaction.

To ease colic, consider eliminating from your diet foods that may cause discomfort to your baby, such as coffee, chocolate, onions, and cruciferous vegetables, including cabbage, broccoli, cauliflower, and Brussels sprouts.

During the first year, it's dangerous to give your baby honey or corn syrup because babies are more vulnerable to botulism. Also, never put anything in a bottle besides breast milk, formula, or water. Nourish your baby with your milk or formula for those first few months until he or she is ready to begin the culinary journey.

PLANT PITFALL

Alcohol passes into breast milk when you drink it. Information is lacking about how much of the alcohol goes into the milk and how long it takes to be metabolized, but know that exposure to alcohol can be detrimental to your baby's development. To be safe, drink no more than one or two servings of alcohol per week while nursing.

Introducing Solids

When your baby starts to show signs that he or she is ready—usually 4 to 6 months of age—it's time to expose your baby's palate to solid foods. (Signs of readiness to start solids include the ability to sit upright and the disappearance of the tongue extrusion reflex. Your baby may also appear curious or interested when watching you eat.)

Supplementing food displaces some of the calories that come from the milk or formula. This is one reason to wait as close to 6 months as possible. Remembering that babies have different nutrient needs, the milk or formula needs to remain the priority of the diet. Think of the solids as accessories and as eating practice.

The first taste adventure to offer is iron-enriched infant cereal. Rice cereal is the best tolerated. Mix in the milk or formula to dilute it at first until your little one develops his or her techniques. Be patient—it takes time to learn how to swallow different textures.

After your baby can take in between $\frac{1}{3}$ and $\frac{1}{2}$ cup cereal, you can begin adding other foods. Keep it to other cereals, fruits, and vegetables for the next few months. Always wait 3 or 4 days after starting one food to introduce a new one so you can monitor for allergies.

 HEALTHY HINT

For years, the AAP recommended against giving highly allergenic foods such as nuts, soy, and wheat to infants until after the age of 2 or even 3. In January 2008, it changed its position, citing inadequate data to delay the introduction of these foods.

Depending on your motivation and your resources, you can make these foods at home, or you can purchase them. Brown rice, oats, and barley can be ground in a blender until very fine and then boiled in water briefly until cooked. Bananas, cooked sweet potatoes, steamed carrots, and avocados can easily be mashed. You can also use pure applesauce, steamed green beans, cooked lentils, and stewed pears.

Use this time to perk up your baby's tastes and preferences. If you start him or her eating close to nature now, you'll provide the best foreground for optimal health in the future.

The Least You Need to Know

- Your diet before conception and through breastfeeding largely impacts your baby's future health.
- During pregnancy, gain the recommended weight to prevent strain on you and your baby.

- Stay consistent with whole-plant foods throughout your pregnancy, and include food sources of DHA, a vitamin B_{12} supplement, and vitamin D and iron if you're deficient.

- You can continue to exercise during pregnancy with a few modifications, as long as you stay tuned in to your body's signals.

- Breastfeeding provides significant health benefits to both you and your baby.

- Solid foods should be slowly and methodically introduced to your little one after the age of 4 to 6 months.

Phyto-Rich Kids

In This Chapter

- Raising a plant-based child
- Fulfilling your little one's nutrient needs
- Feeding picky eaters
- Navigating the school system's diet woes

Approximately 17 percent of children are obese. Puberty is starting earlier in girls than ever before—sometimes as early as age 7—thanks to excess body fat. Early puberty puts our daughters at an increased risk of breast cancer and other chronic diseases later in life. About 2 million adolescents have prediabetes, setting them up for a life plagued with health problems.

Why are our youth so susceptible to these health crises? Partly because they're living sedentary lifestyles. And partly because they're eating most of their calories from animal products and highly processed "foods." The most common fruits and veggies eaten are ketchup and french fries. In a recent USDA survey, only 27 percent of adolescents met daily recommendations for vegetables (3 servings). A mere 15 percent of males and 21 percent of females met the recommended 2 servings of fruits. Whole foods rarely, if ever, touch the lips of most kids on a daily basis. Childhood diet determines future health. The bottom line: we need to fix the food to save our children.

Getting kids to eat healthy can sometimes seem an impossible task. But with a little finesse and some creativity, you can succeed at getting your kids onboard with a plant-based diet.

The Benefits of Growing Up Plant Based

At this point in the book, you know the benefits of following a whole-food, plant-based diet. And if you remember from Chapter 11, the diet consumed during the first decade of a child's life determines his or her health more than the diet of the next 50 years does. Imagine, then, the opportunity you have before you for providing your child with all the nutrients necessary to grow and develop right from the start.

Consider this fascinating example: look at families who move from a rural setting of a non-Western country to an urban, Westernized location. Take rural China, for instance. The older generations who were raised in their homeland on rice, vegetables, fruits, minimal amounts of animal products, and no highly processed foods remain slim and healthy into old age. On the contrary, their children and grandchildren, who have adapted their diets to include fast food, massive amounts of animal products, and highly processed foods, become sick and fat like their new neighbors. Their genes weren't altered on the plane ride to their new home. Their diets changed upon arrival.

Incidence of disease risk differs based on environment. You can't blame your genes. You can, however, change your destiny with the choices you make at each meal.

As a parent, you have control over what your child eats. Until your kids make money and can drive to the store to buy their own food, you're the one bringing home the food. You're the one who can prepare healthy meals. Take full advantage of this opportunity, and set the dietary habits and behaviors that will shape your child's life.

Do as I Say *and* as I Do

The single most important factor determining how your child eats is how *you* eat. Role-modeling is an extremely effective technique for teaching. If you want your kid to love broccoli, Brussels sprouts, lentils, and lima beans, eat them and love them yourself. Do you know how many parents tell their kids to eat their veggies while they themselves fill up on junk food instead? The message it sends is contradicting and confusing. Worse, it doesn't work. You need to be passionate about your food and your health while connecting those dots for your child. When you feel the vitality within your cells, you'll want nothing less for your little one.

Inspire your family by teaching them what you know. Explain that when you eat your leafy greens, your body gets stronger and is able to fight off all the bad germs out there. Eating your beans makes you grow big, with awesome muscles that can lift heavy things. Getting your essential fatty acids makes you so smart, you'll ace all your classes in school.

Make it relevant to your child's life. Excite your child in a language he or she will understand. Of course, this changes throughout childhood, based on where your child's enthusiasm lies and his or her understanding of the world. Your kid is in tune with your feelings and actions, so your best bet for compliance is your own demonstration. Mahatma Gandhi famously suggested, "Be the change you want to see in the world." This axiom applies perfectly to parenthood.

Practice Makes Perfect

As with anything, healthy living takes practice. Learning about the nutrients and how to make nutritious delicious is a work in progress for you and your child. Why not learn and practice together? Use food shopping and cooking as learning experiences.

Spend time in the produce section with your child, talking about the plethora of health-promoting compounds surrounding you. Pick up a tomato and say, "Tomatoes have lycopene, lutein, and vitamin C." Ask your child what you should make for dinner tonight using that tomato. Include him or her in these decisions, because being actively involved infuses passion. When you get home, make the meal together. Even tiny ones can stir, hold things, hand you a spoon, or place items in a pot. The older your child gets, the more capabilities he or she will have. The longer your child is exposed to healthful eating, the deeper his or her understanding and interest will be.

PLANT PITFALL

Gone are the days of the Clean Plate Club. Never push food on your kid. Allow his or her own hunger patterns to emerge without interfering. Hunger changes based on whether it's time for a growth spurt, daily activity, and other factors. Let your child's body be the guide on when it's time to eat and how much.

Experiment with a large variety of foods and recipes, using a few family favorites. Most people rotate among one to three breakfasts, two to four lunches, and five to six dinner options every week. So find what tastes best and is easiest to prepare. Save the more labor-intensive recipes for special occasions.

Keep the options open. Availability of healthy food choices plays a significant role in a child's eating habits. Consider a few tips for increasing access to healthy options:

- Keep a bowl filled with clean, fresh fruits at arm's reach at all times.

- Cut veggies and fruits into bite-size pieces and keep them in the fridge next to healthy dip options (see recipes in Chapter 22).

- Always have a fresh and colorful salad in the fridge with delicious dressings ready to eat.

- Make extra servings when preparing meals so you have leftovers.

- Create your own trail mix with your child. Choose all the nuts, seeds, and dried fruits he or she likes, and package the trail mix in baggies for easy, single-serving treats.

- Stock your cabinets, fridge, and freezer with healthy alternatives so when hunger strikes, you can whip up something fast and easy.

- Make recipes like Figamajigs, Fruity Nut Balls, and AJ's Peanut Bites (recipes in Chapter 23) for quick and satisfying snacks.

Eventually, as your child grows up surrounded by whole-plant foods and knows why you provide these options, a whole-food, plant-based diet will be deeply rooted and more likely to stick. People often warn that when a child gets older, he or she will rebel if the diet is restricted. Rebellion happens as a result of confinement, rigidity, and hefty rules. On the contrary, enthusiasm, knowledge, and room for variety simply lead to habit. It's well established that people develop behavior based on what they learn at home. Fortunately, then, it's in your hands: create the soil you want your child's roots to grow in.

PLANT PITFALL

Don't reward or bribe your kid with food or punish him or her by taking away certain foods. This adds a psychological component to food, which can affect your child later in life. Find other ways to motivate instead.

Meeting Their Macro- and Micronutrient Needs

When it comes to recommendations for what children need nutrition-wise, charts and lists from medical and government authorities abound. Their recommendations include how many servings per day from each food group, percentage of saturated fat as a maximum, and advice on taking the skin off the chicken before eating it.

Somehow, though, this information isn't translating. Parents aren't paying attention. Fast food is a daily meal for about one third of youths. That means one in three children eats fast food every single day! No matter how "happy" or "healthy" the option is at a fast-food establishment, it's impossible to achieve proper nutrient recommendations or avoid the mass quantities of saturated fat, cholesterol, and animal protein in these meals. In addition, the "food" is as processed as possible and as far away from nature as anything edible.

The two places where nutrition is most important—schools and hospitals—often serve the least nutritious food. Have you seen what the school cafeteria serves for lunch these days? The government-subsidized commodities are typically huge boxes of ground meats and cheeses. When the school receives its shipment, it gets to decide what to make with the items to serve the kids. Many hospitals now house fast-food chains inside their buildings. Furthermore, junk food has replaced real food in lunch boxes, in school cafeteria lunch lines, at parties, for sports practices, and at other events.

MIXED GREENS

Excuses for why fast food and junk food have become so prevalent include no time to cook and not enough money to afford healthy options. But these excuses fall short when you actually analyze the possibilities. Opening a can of beans and a jar of salsa and warming some corn tortillas in the oven takes less time than stopping at a fast-food restaurant drive-thru. Batch cooking is even more cost- and time-efficient: buy foods in bulk (whole grains, beans, seeds, nuts, and spices) and prepare large amounts at the same time. Package, freeze, and reheat when it's dinnertime.

You may be wondering what kids need to be healthy. Overall, they need the same thing you need to be healthy: a wide assortment of vegetables, fruits, whole grains, legumes, nuts, and seeds. Encourage and challenge your child to eat every color of the rainbow each day as a way of increasing variety. If you emphasize and provide these foods, you can easily meet all your child's nutrient needs (except for vitamin B_{12} and possibly vitamin D).

Generally, macronutrient needs can be met with adequate calorie intake, and if you give your child the freedom to eat whenever he or she feels hungry, calorie needs will automatically be fulfilled. If you provide whole-food options at those times of hunger, macronutrient and micronutrient needs will both be met. The body is naturally self-regulating and adjusts according to activity levels and periods of growth.

Don't forget the vitamins B_{12} and D. All herbivores, regardless of age, need to supplement with vitamin B_{12}. And all people—herbivore or omnivore—need to be tested for vitamin D levels and treated if deficient. Breastfed infants should be given 400 IU vitamin D as a supplement, because their sun exposure is usually inadequate and breast milk doesn't provide enough vitamin D. The adequate intake for vitamin D is 200 IU per day. However, if blood levels fall below 30 ng/mL, it's necessary to supplement. In this case, ask your pediatrician to recommend the proper dosage.

The following table lists the recommendations for vitamin B_{12} for various ages.

Vitamin B_{12} Requirements for Children

Age	Daily Requirement (mcg)
1 to 3 years	0.9
4 to 8 years	1.2
9 to 13 years	1.8
14 years and up	2.4

Pleasing Picky Palates

Kids are picky eaters—and that's when they're eating everything under the sun. You might be wondering how you'll ever succeed in trying to feed them a whole-food, plant-based diet.

This scenario might sound familiar: your kid's hungry, so you try to feed him something nutritious. He doesn't like it and protests, asking for something not so healthy. You persist. Next comes the whining or tantrum-throwing (your child, not you—although you might feel like throwing a tantrum!). Finally, you give in.

This episode is common in parenting, especially with toddlers and preschoolers. The biggest problem stemming from this scenario is its self-perpetuating nature. Your child learns that whining, screaming, or begging (or all of the above) eventually works.

As I mentioned in Chapter 6, if you're not hungry enough to eat an apple, you're probably not really hungry. The same goes for your little one. Don't be afraid that your child won't get enough food to eat. Remember that kid-size bodies are smaller than yours and don't always need as many calories. Also, when your child is hungry, he or she will eat. Kids won't let themselves starve. If you try force-feeding just to calm your concern, you're only setting yourself up for frustration.

Many kids get stuck on a mono diet, only wanting to choose among a few staples. Although this can be disconcerting to a concerned parent, some simple strategies may help. First and foremost, be the master of your kitchen. Stock only the foods you want your family to eat. Also, provide variations at each meal and snack. For instance, my kids are obsessed with pasta and request it for dinner daily. I switch it up by alternating among corn, whole-wheat, rice, and quinoa noodles each night so they're exposed to different grains. I also change up what I add to the pasta. Some nights, they find broccoli and peas in their pasta, and other nights, it's kale and lima beans.

One strategy you may try is to implement the "one-bite rule." Make it a rule that your child must taste one bite of a new food you're offering before deciding he or she doesn't like it. Stay the course, and be consistent in offering a variety of options. If your child is truly hungry, he or she will eat what you have to offer. Eventually this phase ends anyway, and your child's palate will expand.

HEALTHY HINT

Creativity counts big time with kids! Using fun names and making animals or different characters out of fruits and veggies goes a long way toward making food exciting. Think ants on a log (celery with nut butter and raisins on top), banana boats (bananas cut lengthwise and filled with nut butter, hempseeds, and dried fruit), and chocolate smoothies (with leafy greens, dates, almond milk, raw cocoa powder, and frozen fruit). Use cookie cutters to stamp out fun shapes for healthy sandwiches or whole-food cookies. Use seaweed, collard greens, or whole-grain tortillas to make fancy wraps.

Another issue is food addiction. Depending on your child's age when you introduce whole foods, those taste buds may already be distorted. Regularly eating sugar, oil, and salt causes food addiction even at a young age. However, explaining the science to your little one will be senseless and not helpful. Thus, you need to be persistent, especially at the beginning of the transition. Prepare the majority of meals and snacks at home. It's already hard enough to protect your kid from junk food at school and parties, so try to have whole-food options in every other situation. Soon enough, taste buds will improve, addiction will subside, and whole foods will be appealing.

Surviving School

Schools are nutritional wastelands. With the National School Lunch Program, the School Breakfast Program, and the vast overavailability of junk food at every opportunity, you have to put on your power parenting skills to fight off the antinutrients.

Meeting government standards for the nutrient levels in the school food meals is bad enough, but when I spent some time in school food service during my dietetic internship, I was advised to increase the quantity of ketchup used in an average meal so the computer analysis would show a lower total fat percentage of calories. (Apparently, ketchup really is a fruit or vegetable serving in the school world.) The requirements themselves are lenient enough; still, the actual intake numbers need to be exaggerated to appear to meet the standards.

Moreover, when produce is offered—in the form of salad bars, for instance—the presentation is unappealing and drab sitting right next to the brightly packaged chips, sugary products, and deeply fried reheated foods. If given those choices, which would you choose?

Furthermore, schools are still required to offer kids milk—even if the cartons are chocolate or strawberry milk at every meal. Oddly, dairy-free options are seldom, if ever, provided. No wonder the number of kids diagnosed with ADD, ADHD, obesity, and other more serious health complications is growing!

MIXED GREENS

The Dietary Guidelines for Americans is the basis for menu planning in the school system. Therefore, school lunches are required to meet only the standard of no more than 30 percent total calories from fat and less than 10 percent from saturated fat. Also, the school needs only offer one third of the RDAs for vitamin A, vitamin C, iron, calcium, and total calories.

What can a concerned parent do to avoid getting absorbed into this misguided, disease-promoting arrangement? Most important, pack your child's school lunch every day. Send healthy choices like you would provide at home, and include special treats to prevent curiosity and desire to buy food at school. Maximize your creativity here so your little one enjoys his or her lunch and doesn't feel left out.

Here are some ideas for yummy, nutrient-dense lunchbox items:

- Sprouted- or whole-grain bread with almond, cashew, or peanut butter and pure fruit spread or sliced bananas
- Sprouted- or whole-grain bread with hummus and sliced cucumbers and tomatoes
- Sushi rolls made with brown rice, cucumbers, avocado, and carrots
- Noritos (recipe in Chapter 20)
- Sweet Pea Guacamole (recipe in Chapter 22) with baked tortilla chips
- Homemade trail mix your child helped make with his or her favorite nuts, seeds, and dried fruits
- Figamajigs (recipe in Chapter 23)
- Pineapple, peach, apple, or pear chunks
- Large, pitted olives
- Fresh fruit with a nut butter or date syrup dipping sauce
- Veggie pizza on whole-grain crust with pineapple, olives, mushrooms, and/or bell peppers
- Oil-free, salt-free popcorn with nutritional yeast sprinkled on top
- Simply Hummus (recipe in Chapter 22) with raw, chopped veggies (cherry or grape tomatoes, baby carrots, sugar snap peas, jicama sticks, button mushrooms, celery sticks, baby corn, blanched green beans, or blanched asparagus spears)
- Unclassic Oatmeal Raisin Cookies (recipe in Chapter 23)

Additionally, be active in the planning committees at school. Get involved in arranging class parties and events where food is involved. Argue your points with detailed facts to encourage the other parents, school faculty, and teachers to make healthier decisions. The louder your squeaky wheel, the more likely they'll listen and learn.

Finally, write letters including statistics and health information to your school; school district; and local, state, and national government officials. As a concerned and impassioned parent and citizen, you have a voice.

If we are to improve the state of our children's health, changes must be implemented. We are currently sliding downhill fast, and if we don't provide our kids with nutritious options at each meal, they'll only continue to fall. This generation is the first in recorded history predicted to live a shorter lifespan than the preceding generation. What does that tell you about our state of health? Take action to protect your child—loudly and backed up with facts. The only thing you have to lose is the health of your most precious commodity.

Start at home, where you have total control, and branch out. Build your case by showing fellow parents the results of eating a nutrient-dense lifestyle: less sickness; improved performance in school (both academically and athletically); and happy, healthy kids. Be the role model for your child and for other parents, and change will come.

The Least You Need to Know

- Growing up on a whole-food, plant-based diet sets the foundation for lifelong optimal health.
- Be the change you want to see in your child. Role-modeling is the most effective tool for inspiring and teaching healthy eating.
- Let your child gauge his or her own hunger. Children won't let themselves starve.
- Always have whole-plant options available in the house and when on the go.
- Supplement your little one's whole-food, plant-based diet with vitamin B_{12} and, if he or she's deficient, vitamin D.
- Survive school's nutritional wasteland by sending lunch to school, participating in activity planning, and being vocal about why and how to provide healthier options.

Super-Plant Seniors

In This Chapter

- Staying vital and active in your golden years
- Nutrient changes as you age
- Dealing with physical obstacles associated with aging
- Keeping your kitchen simple
- Managing medication complications

The secrets to aging gracefully are surfacing, with more evidence supporting the benefits of healthy living. After recently spending time visiting a relative in a nursing home, the desperate need for reformed health management became even more blaringly obvious to me. What's the point of living well into old age if you're not able to enjoy it? With medical advances, people can be kept alive by invasive procedures and strong medications for decades. Unfortunately, these advancements come with a price.

The good news is it's never too late to start taking care of your body. Living a healthy lifestyle can help keep you active and youthful while avoiding cardiovascular disease, diabetes, osteoporosis, arthritis, obesity, and most cancers. A whole-food, plant-based diet—together with exercise, adequate sleep, and stress management—appears to be that fountain of youth we've all been searching for.

Living Larger, Longer

It might sound strange, but we should all strive for a natural death. Physicians say leading a vital, active life well into old age until you simply slip painlessly away is the best plan for living. Many people object to this idea, arguing that a shorter life is preferential to overhauling diet and lifestyle. Unfortunately, the choice isn't that simple. Quality of life and functional independence matter most; these objectives are precisely what you can control with your lifestyle choices.

Although how *long* you live comes with no guarantees, eating well, exercising consistently, and managing stress improves how *great* you live and how long you maintain your youth. The story of World Strongman Joe Rollino epitomizes this point: Joe ate a vegetarian diet while abstaining from cigarettes and alcohol. Considered one of the greatest performing strongmen ever to live, he recently, at the age of 104, was killed when hit by a car during his daily 5-mile walk. Although his story is ironic, it demonstrates that lifestyle leads to vitality and health, even in your centenarian years.

MIXED GREENS

Current life expectancy at birth is 77.9 years. The oldest documented person was a French woman who lived to the age of 122 years and 164 days. Life expectancy is higher in non-meat-eaters than meat-eaters. Vegetarians live about 7 years longer, and vegans live 15 years longer than meat-eaters.

Typically, after a lifetime of eating poorly and remaining sedentary, the cardiovascular system breaks down. Vascular events occur either at powerful enough levels to induce death (as in a massive heart attack or stroke) or at small degrees, which can lead to dementia, blood clots, and minimized freedom of movement. In the case of the latter, seniors can survive for many years with medications that lower blood pressure and cholesterol, stent placements in their arteries, or bypass surgeries. They may be kept alive, but are they really living? Suffering with illness heavily influences daily life. Visiting doctors or enduring tests and procedures isn't the same as traveling, taking dancing lessons, or enjoying time with people you love.

In the nursing home environment, most residents sit around in wheelchairs or lie in their beds for most of the day. Yet our bodies have the potential for so much more than this scenario. You can find plenty of wonderful examples of fit, healthy seniors living joyously active lives. With some simple lifestyle tweaks, you can enrich your senior years and extend your capacity for deliciously living well into old age. Be defiant. Redefine the meaning of aging gracefully.

Naturally Enhanced Nutrient Needs

Your nutrient requirements change throughout your lifespan. Your need for many micronutrients increases after age 51 and then again after age 70. Adding to the challenge of meeting these increased needs is the fact that most people eat less as they grow older. This means you must focus on nutrient density and make every bite count.

Your metabolism slows as you age because of muscle loss, decreased physical activity, and reduced digestion efficiency. Therefore, to maintain your ideal body weight, you need to eat fewer calories. The metabolism myth presented in Chapter 6 explains why the less you eat, the slower you age. Ideally, you need to make your diet so nutrient-dense that you can get away with eating only as much as your body truly needs.

HEALTHY HINT

Muscle mass declines by approximately 1 percent per year after age 40. On average, you lose 30 percent of your strength between age 50 and 70, and then another 30 percent each decade after that. Exercise combats this loss, helping you maintain muscle strength and function. Incorporating strength training a few times a week is an excellent investment in your quality of life. It's never too late to start!

Your calcium and vitamin B_6 requirements increase slightly after age 51, so to enhance your intake, emphasize leafy green vegetables, broccoli, baked potatoes, bananas, oats, tofu, beans, and seeds. Circulating vitamin D levels in the blood decrease as you grow older, especially after age 70. As with every other age group, continue to stay on top of your 25-hydroxyvitamin D blood test and supplement as necessary.

Because of the higher risk of osteoporosis and fractures in advanced age, it's critical to maintain optimum levels of vitamin D and calcium. Supplement with D if your blood test reveals suboptimal levels, and eat plenty of calcium-rich plant foods.

Iron is harmful in excess amounts because it induces oxidation. Once women reach menopause, they stop losing iron via their monthly menstrual cycle and their iron requirements return to those of the prepuberty years to prevent overconsumption. Supplementation is necessary only as a stop-gap measure to address a deficiency for a temporary period of time. Usually, an iron deficiency indicates a medical problem instead of a nutritional imbalance.

Vitamin B$_{12}$ deficiency is extremely common among the elderly, regardless of diet. A common condition called *atrophic gastritis* is often to blame, as are depleted vitamin B$_{12}$ stores, insufficient intake, and inadequate absorption. So be sure to consume adequate amounts of foods fortified with B$_{12}$ (plant milks and nutritional yeast are excellent options) and take a supplement of 5 to 10 micrograms a day.

DEFINITION

Atrophic gastritis is chronic inflammation of the stomach lining that interferes with vitamin B$_{12}$ absorption. It affects up to half of adults over age 60.

The following tables list the recommendations for micronutrients for both men and women at various ages.

Micronutrient Needs for Older Men

Nutrient	Age 31 to 50	Age 51 to 70	Age 70 and Over
Vitamin B$_6$	1.3mg	1.7mg	1.7mg
Vitamin D	5mcg	10mcg	15mcg
Calcium	1,000mg	1,200mg	1,200mg
Iron	14mg	14mg	14mg

Micronutrient Needs for Older Women

Nutrient	Age 31 to 50	Age 51 to 70	Age 70 and Over
Vitamin B$_6$	1.3mg	1.5mg	1.5mg
Vitamin D	5mcg	10mcg	15mcg
Calcium	1,000mg	1,200mg	1,200mg
Iron	33mg	14mg	14mg

Dealing with Age-Related Physical Changes

Seniors have unique challenges when it comes to eating optimally. Malnutrition is common, due to multiple factors. Many medications and chronic conditions affect appetite, hydration, swallowing, digestion, and/or absorption. Naturally occurring physical changes of aging, like decreased appetite, chewing difficulty, decreased taste sensation, mobility limitations, and sluggish GI function, also impact food consumption. Psychological factors come into play as well. Depression, fatigue, loneliness, anxiety, and cognitive decline are common and make eating choices less of a priority.

Ideally, eating a nutrient-rich, plant-based diet prevents many of these issues. Chronic conditions that elicit the need for medications should not exist, and limitations of movement capacity should not occur. The lifelong neglect of proactive nourishment and adequate exercise is what leads to these problems. However, if you find yourself struggling with challenges, establish a solid plan to help you get the nutrients necessary to improve your health.

HEALTHY HINT

Constipation is common in older adults, thanks to sluggish digestion, medications, and inadequate food intake. Concentrate on consuming high-fiber foods like beans, whole grains, vegetables, and fruits every day, and get plenty of fluids.

Dealing with Your Diet

The more prepared you are to prepare whole, plant-based foods, the more likely you are to actually do so. If necessary, enlist the help of your friends and/or family, to be sure you have all the resources you need at your fingertips.

Stock your kitchen with user-friendly equipment, such as a high-powered blender, rice cooker/steamer, slow cooker, automatic can opener, and pots and pans. Fill your pantry, fridge, and freezer with your favorite healthy options. If someone can help you do your shopping, you can buy more items at once. If not, simply make going to the store a part of your routine to pick up items you need for that day.

To simplify food preparation, keep frozen fruits, vegetables, and brown rice handy at all times. Frozen veggie burgers come in handy for a quick meal. Canned beans without added salt are great to include in at least one meal a day. Also stock your pantry with the following (along with a jar opener to assist you):

- Canned tomatoes
- Jars of olives and crushed garlic
- Sprouted whole-grain pasta
- Whole grains—oats, brown rice, quinoa, barley

- Dried lentils

- Raw nuts and seeds

- Fortified plant-based milks

- Low-sodium vegetable broths and other soup blends

- Corn or rice cakes

- Whole-grain crackers

When you prepare an extra serving or two to eat the following day, you don't have to cook every day. Use recipes you're comfortable with, as long as they're nutrient-dense. If they're not, add color and substitute whole-food versions of the original ingredients. For instance, if your favorite dinner is pasta marinara, choose whole-grain pasta and oil-free marinara sauce, and stir in chopped broccoli and kale.

Many simple meals don't take too much time or effort. Keep your focus on easy. To save time, you can buy nutritious prepared foods at your local health food store or restaurant. Always seek out color, especially green, and other items that follow the recommendations in this book. And be sure to choose wisely, because you need to maximize nutrient intake for the least amount of calories to stay healthy.

Dealing with Medicine Mayhem

For many seniors, with the passage of years comes the addition of new medications to the daily regimen. As the chronic conditions pile up, so do the prescriptions. Unfortunately, the vast majority of doctors prefer to assign a condition or symptom to a pill instead of digging into the patient's lifestyle. When was the last time your doctor asked you what you eat and whether you exercise? If your doctor does that, keep him or her, and refer all your friends!

PLANT PITFALL

Polypharmacy, the use of multiple medications, is a risk to your overall health. Many medications interact with other ones by increasing or decreasing the effects or causing side effects. Be sure to tell each one of your doctors exactly which pills you're taking, including any supplements, herbs, tonics, or elixirs. Always keep a list handy when you go to an appointment.

The main reason for this prescription-obsessed epidemic is that medical school teaches precisely that—how to find the perfect pill to fix or at least quiet the symptom. Major changes to medical school curriculum, government regulations, and separation of drug companies from physician education are critical. Until these changes come to fruition, you have to look out for yourself. Doing things like reading this book and implementing my recommendations will help you live long and large.

Please know that medical care is extremely advantageous—especially in certain situations—but there's a whole world out there beyond pill popping and symptom soothing. If your body is reacting with high blood pressure, for example, something bigger is wrong, and you need to address the issue. Most of the time, a majority of indications are diet related and can be alleviated by switching to a whole-food, plant-based diet.

Certain medications interact with foods. A common example is the drug Warfarin, or Coumadin, and vitamin K. Warfarin is a drug commonly prescribed to thin the blood and prevent clotting. Vitamin K naturally helps the liver make blood-clotting factors. Taking Warfarin prevents the liver from taking this action. You might be wondering how this interaction affects you if you're taking this medication. Consistency in your vitamin K consumption is vitally important. If you eat too many vitamin K–rich foods, you decrease the effect of the Warfarin. Conversely, if you eat fewer vitamin K–rich foods, you increase the blood-thinning effect of Warfarin.

Leafy green vegetables are the highest in vitamin K. Kale has the most, with 547 micrograms per cup, raw. Spinach, collard greens, broccoli, and chard are also rich sources. This doesn't mean you shouldn't eat these foods if you take Warfarin; just maintain a consistent amount every day to prevent fluctuations in the effectiveness of the drug.

Here are some other points to consider with respect to medications:

- All drugs have side effects.
- Be vocal with your physician about any reactions you have to your medications, to be sure your dose and the type of drug is appropriate.
- Bring up diet with your doctor, and ask if you need to be concerned about any food-drug interactions with your current prescriptions.

As you transition to a whole-food, plant-based diet, be sure you tell your doctor to supervise your medications carefully. Most people reduce or eliminate their need for their meds as their body naturally begins to heal. With drugs such as those that lower insulin or blood pressure, not monitoring carefully can be life-threatening. For example, changing your diet helps lower your blood pressure. If you remain on the dosage you started with, your blood pressure can end up too low and cause you to pass out.

The good news is that if you and your doctor are vigilant about monitoring and following the guidelines presented in this book, you have a good chance of getting off your current medications.

The Least You Need to Know

- Eating a whole-food, plant-based diet and exercising regularly can help ward off the chronic illnesses and physical disabilities common in the later years.
- Nutrient density is critical to your diet later in life. Metabolism slows naturally, but you still need to consume all the necessary nutrients.
- Slow the aging process by eating efficiently—high amounts of micronutrients with fewer macronutrients.
- Micronutrient needs for vitamin B_6, vitamin D, and calcium increase after age 50. Seniors also must be vigilant about getting adequate vitamin B_{12} daily.
- Tell all your doctors about all your medications and supplements, and ask about possible interactions, including potential reactions with foods.
- If you're transitioning to a whole-food, plant-based diet after being on medications (especially meds that lower insulin or blood pressure), have your doctor monitor you closely for any needed adjustments.

Plant-Strong Athletes

In This Chapter

- Enhancing your performance with plant-based fuel
- The importance of timing with nutrients
- Tips for staying hydrated
- Dispelling myths about performance enhancers

Nobody requires perfect nutrition like an athlete does. As an athlete, the food you choose to fuel your body can give you an extra edge to separate you from the pack. And whole-food, plant-based nutrition gives you what you need to push your body to its maximum intensity.

Elite athletes from many different sports have demonstrated the advantages of going plant-based in their training and performance. And from what we've seen, the results of a plant-based nutrition plan are phenomenal.

Ultramarathoner Grant Campbell says, "On a plant-based diet, I can run 60 miles through mountains and enjoy running again the next day; running injuries don't haunt me anymore; and I never lose training time because I never get sick." And Carl Lewis, winner of 10 Olympic medals (9 golds) and 10 World Championship medals, is quoted as saying that his best performances came when he was 30 years old and vegan. In this chapter, you learn how you, too, can find success as a plant-based athlete.

Bringing Your "A" Game with Plants

The premise of exercise is muscle tissue breakdown. Any physical stress you place on your body causes microscopic tears in your muscle tissue. The tougher the workout, the more damage to your muscles. The post-exercise period is the critical period when all the recovering, rebuilding, and replenishing takes place. At this point, providing optimal and varied nutrients that your body can easily absorb is especially significant. This period between workouts and performances determines your improvements. If you fuel yourself properly and get adequate sleep and rest, your muscles will build back stronger than before, ready to perform more efficiently next time.

> **HEALTHY HINT**
>
> The breaking down of muscle tissue is called catabolism, and the building back up is called anabolism. Both are constantly occurring throughout your body. To maximize strength, power, endurance, and agility, you want the anabolism to overpower the catabolism. Do this by emphasizing adequate and proper fuel.

Whole-plant foods provide an extra benefit because of nutrient density; plants provide a huge variety of both the macronutrients and micronutrients your body thrives on. Remember from Chapter 4 that exercise causes an increase in the presence of free radicals. This means antioxidants are required at higher levels to alleviate the stress placed on your body. The best sources for antioxidants and free radical–fighting phytochemicals are whole fruits and vegetables.

In addition, you need a lot of energy to fuel performance. Processed foods and animal products provide empty calories that take up space in your digestive tract and bloodstream; a better plan is to consume actively beneficial foods. Top-level athletes from track and field, bodybuilding, triathlons, football, mixed martial arts, cycling, baseball, ice hockey, basketball, tennis, boxing, and more have incorporated—and set records with—a plant-based diet.

Macronutrient Needs for Athletes

Sports nutrition is a unique specialty, traditionally focused on calculating the appropriate macronutrient intakes at the right times. The basis is in quantifying, counting, and measuring. Of course, you need a proper amount of carbs, protein, and fat to fuel performance and recover effectively. But let's take this a step—or mile—farther.

With plant-based sports nutrition, you can broaden your body's capabilities by carefully selecting where those macronutrients come from. Not all foods are treated equally after you swallow them. From digestion and absorption all the way to how your body utilizes them when they're in the bloodstream, nutrients act differently based on their source. When you're applying these nutrients to a body pushing itself to extremes with training and performance, the difference in fuel choice becomes apparent. Why give your car regular gasoline if it costs the same to choose high-octane fuel—especially if you'll get enhanced performance?

Certain foods are easier on your system, providing an alkalizing effect on your body and focusing your energy on performance instead of stressful digestion. Just as a day has only 24 hours, you have a limited capacity for energy. As an athlete, you need to use your energy efficiently. Selecting foods that steal energy from performance and recovery is wasteful and ineffective. Alternatively, eating whole-plant foods at the right times can take your performance to new heights.

MIXED GREENS

Some famous plant-based athletes include track and field Olympian Carl Lewis, tennis player Martina Navratilova, mixed martial artist Mac Danzig, ultramarathoner Scott Jurek, NFL tight end Tony Gonzalez, boxer Keith Holmes, Ironman triathlete Brendan Brazier, ultramarathoner Grant Campbell, ice hockey player Georges Laraque, triathlete Ruth Heidrich, bodybuilder Robert Hazeley, NFL wide receiver Desmond Howard, and bodybuilder Robert Cheeke.

One of the most important factors in sports nutrition—besides the quality of your food choices—is adequate intake. Depending on your activity level, sport, and individual metabolic needs, you need to monitor closely how much you consume. Exercising at high intensity, frequency, and duration requires a lot of calories. Ultimately, your macronutrient needs are the same, but you need more of them overall. Instead of using a generic formula to determine how many calories you need, follow this simple protocol:

- Eat when you're hungry.

- Choose high-quality plant foods.

- Carefully plan your intake around your training (see the "Nutrient Timing" section, later in this chapter).

- Monitor your weight. If you're at your ideal weight for your performance demands, maintain it. If you're losing weight, you're not eating enough. If you're gaining weight, either eat less or reassess the composition of your food choices.

Just as in everyday healthy life, your body knows better than any formula. Listen to your signals—hunger and satiation as well as performance—to determine what *you* need.

Carbohydrates as Fuel and for Recovery

Carbs are the most efficient source of fuel. With respect to sports, the difference between simple and complex carbs is crucial. Simple carbs are digested quickly and end up in the bloodstream faster than any other macronutrient, providing nearly instantaneous energy. These are your best friends when it comes to preworkout meals, intake during endurance exercise, and replenishment immediately after exercise. Complex carbs are slower to absorb, thanks to their fiber content. Consume these the evening before an event and a couple hours before training or performance to give you sustainability.

Carbs are stored in your body, in your muscles and your liver, as glycogen. (Two thirds to three fourths is stored in your muscles, and the rest is stored in your liver.) During exercise, you first use up the glucose circulating in your blood. Next, you start breaking down the stored glycogen to provide more glucose for immediate use. After you use up your stored glycogen, you run out of fuel and need to replenish. And the more trained you are, the more your body is able to use stored fat for energy. This spares glycogen use and improves endurance.

Because of their easy digestibility, simple carbs are the best choices to consume just before exercising. Excellent sources of simple carbs include fresh fruits, dried fruits (especially dates), and green smoothies.

Complex carbs have more fiber, which can cause cramps or discomfort, taking away energy from where it should be—your muscles. After your workout or performance, complex carbs are perfect to help refill your glycogen reserves so you can prepare for next time. Excellent sources of complex carbs include whole grains (brown rice, oats, barley, quinoa), potatoes, sweet potatoes, yams, corn, whole-grain pasta, sprouted bread or tortillas, beans, and lentils.

PLANT PITFALL

Never try anything new before a game, race, or performance. Practice what you eat and drink—and the timing in which you do so—beforehand to prevent a negative response.

Muscle: Gym-Built, Not Kitchen-Made

Protein plays a huge role in post-exercise recovery and the rebuilding process. Your body requires protein to create muscle tissue, hormones, enzymes, ligaments, tendons, and cells. Consuming adequate amounts helps maintain the circulating pool of amino acids, supporting fluid balance, and proper acid-base equilibrium. Immune function holds steady with proper protein replenishment. But is more necessarily better? If you consume huge levels of protein, will you recover better or build bigger muscles? No. More intake usually does not equal more results.

Your body works on a careful balance beam, always striving to maintain homeostasis. If you consume too much of anything, your body works to fit it into your cells. If you don't need something, your body either stores the excess or disposes of it. You can't fool your ingenious body. If you want big muscles, work out properly in the gym. If you want increased strength, train appropriately. If you want to be faster, learn the drills to train smart.

In most sports, excessive protein consumption is considered an advantage. Yet the research suggesting any benefit is unproven. From what we know about the harms of high protein intakes, especially from animal sources, you may be putting your body at risk for long-term damage by following this suggestion. Interestingly, because athletes require more calories, you automatically get more protein when you eat more food. Selecting whole, unprocessed plant foods makes it impossible not to meet adequate protein requirements.

Hundreds, if not thousands, of protein powders, drinks, bars, and supplements are currently on the market. These are notoriously full of milk-based whey protein plus fillers, stabilizers, preservatives, sweeteners, flavors, and other compounds that wreak havoc on your body. They cost a lot of money and promise you the perfect body or ultimate performance. Yet due to the guidelines set by the Dietary Supplement Health and Education Act, manufacturers are allowed to make such health claims on the packages as "burns fat instead of storing it," "designed exactly to the needs of human metabolism," or "supplies highest quality amino acids." As tempting as these promises sound, nobody has to prove they're truthful. Nor does anyone have to prove long-term safety of their use. So if these products don't work, they're expensive, and they can potentially be harmful, what's the point?

Nutrient Timing

Believe it or not, *when* you eat and drink surrounding exercise can be just as important as *what* you eat. Fueling and recovering your body in a strategic manner benefits your performance.

In this section, I break down some general guidelines, but you know your body and how it functions best. Part of your training focus needs to be on which foods and drinks offer the most advantage, as well as when you consume them. Practice makes perfect. Experiment until you know with precision what your body requires to thrive.

MIXED GREENS

Professional Ironman triathlete and author Brendan Brazier says, "Quick recovery is the key to athletic success. 80% of the recovery process can be attributed to nutrition."

Eating and hydrating before exercise improves your performance, although you don't want to force your body to focus on digestion by filling up too much. Here are some tips for success:

- Eat something small that's high in easily digestible carbs and low in fiber, protein, and fat 90 minutes to 2 hours before your event.

- Drink 1 or 2 cups fluid—preferably a beverage including 6 to 8 percent carbohydrates—1 hour before an event.

- Make good choices such as fruits (dried or fresh), a bagel with whole-fruit jam or fruit "butter," or a plant-based fruit yogurt.

During an event lasting an hour, sports drinks are helpful, especially if the event occurs first thing in the morning after an overnight fast. For events longer than 1 hour, keep the following in mind:

- Maintain hydration by sipping water and sports drinks with 6 to 8 percent carbs consistently throughout the event.

- Consume carbs in the form of sports gels, bars, or drinks at 15- to 20-minute intervals.

- Consume 0.7 grams of carbs per kilogram of body weight per hour (approximately 30 to 60 grams per hour) to improve endurance.

Immediately after an event, a magical window of opportunity opens during which your body is ready, willing, and eager to absorb nourishment. Within 30 to 45 minutes after finishing is the most critical time to replenish stores. Your muscles are able to soak up the glycogen at an increased rate during this time. Plus, you need to refill the antioxidant stores you used up. During this opportunity, choose foods that are …

- High in simple carbs, so they're absorbed as soon as possible.

- Low in fat without too much fiber, because those slow digestion.

- Low in protein at a ratio of 1 part protein to 4 parts carbs, to help speed glycogen synthesis.

Excellent post-event choices include these:

- A green smoothie with lots of fruits, leafy greens, and coconut water

- Whole-grain pasta with oil-free marinara sauce

- Quinoa with vegetables

- Stir-fry with brown rice and veggies

- Veggie sushi

Whole-y Hydration

Proper hydration during exercise is critical for performance and for your safety. Dehydration, a loss of 2 percent of your body weight from fluids, can compromise your performance; impair your mental function; and even lead to serious, life-threatening consequences. Signs of dehydration include muscle cramps, spasms, decreased performance, thirst, and diminishing rate of sweat.

You lose fluids and *electrolytes* at increased levels during exercise, thanks to your increased breathing rate and sweat. Depending on the duration, the intensity, your fitness level, and the weather, the amount of fluid and electrolyte you need varies.

Preventing Dehydration and Hyponatremia

Normally, your body is extremely proficient at maintaining proper electrolyte balance. Slight fluctuations occur, but a drastic shift can have life-threatening consequences.

People with kidney disease or those who take certain medications can experience problems balancing electrolytes. However, certain behaviors can cause an imbalance as well. Consuming large amounts of water without also taking in sodium can cause a condition known as *hyponatremia*, which can cause confusion, drowsiness, muscle weakness, nausea, vomiting, brain swelling, headaches, twitches, and seizures. To prevent hyponatremia, don't overhydrate before an event or rely on water as your sole fluid source during endurance events.

DEFINITION

Electrolytes are minerals found in the blood that help balance fluids and maintain normal functions like your heart's rhythm and muscle contraction. The main electrolytes are sodium, potassium, chloride, magnesium, calcium, phosphate, and bicarbonate. **Hyponatremia** is an abnormally low concentration of sodium in the blood (less than 130 mEq per liter) that can cause cells to malfunction and can be fatal. It can result from prolonged, heavy sweating with failure to replenish sodium or from excessive water consumption, so it has become common in high-endurance athletes.

Follow these tips on maintaining proper hydration:

- At least 4 hours before you exercise, drink 2 or 3 milliliters of water per pound of body weight to optimize hydration status.

- Because fluid needs vary greatly during exercise, you can determine your fluid requirements by routinely measuring your body weight before and after training. Weighing yourself before and after exercise can help you learn how to prevent a loss of 2 pounds over the course of the session.

- Generally, try to take in about 4 to 8 ounces ($\frac{1}{2}$ to 1 cup) of fluids every 20 minutes during exercise.

- For exercise events lasting longer than an hour, drink beverages containing 6 to 8 percent of calories from carbohydrates.

- After exercise, drink 2 or 3 cups of fluid for every pound of body weight lost.

Sports Drinks: What Type and When?

For events lasting longer than 90 minutes, sports drinks with carbs and electrolytes help spare glycogen, prevent dehydration and hyponatremia, and maintain electrolyte balance.

Several varieties are commercially available, but most of them contain large amounts of sugar, artificial colors, and artificial flavors. Instead, you can substitute coconut water or make your own sports beverage with diluted 100 percent pure fruit juice and a touch of sea salt.

Ergogenic Aids

Ergogenic aids, nutritional products that enhance performance, are widely used in the athletic community. No matter what promises the labels claim, very few of them are effective.

No pill, powder, or supplement can produce the same results as hard work and consistency in training. Worse, many of them are dangerous to your health. And some are against the rules. National and international sports organizations monitor for certain ergogenic aids with random urine testing to prevent their use in competitions.

Pushing your body to the ultimate extreme is the essence of athleticism. This population, more than any other, requires optimal nutrition to succeed in performance and recovery. Careful attention to nutrient timing and consistent hydration takes your body and your results beyond what you thought possible as an athlete. If maintaining a whole-food, plant-based diet is effective when challenging your body at its maximum capacity, it represents the potential for every body to be plant-strong.

The Least You Need to Know

- Athletes require optimal nutrition because their bodies are constantly breaking down and rebuilding cells. Eating a whole-food, plant-based diet can take your performance to the next level.
- As an athlete, you don't need extra protein or different ratios of carbs, proteins, and fats. Eating enough calories from high-quality, whole-plant foods naturally provides what your body requires.
- Simple carbs provide excellent fuel both before and during workouts, as well as give you post-workout replenishment.
- Eat within 30 to 45 minutes of finishing an event or training to take advantage of the superabsorption window of opportunity.
- Proper hydration not only drastically impacts performance but is also critical for your safety. Stay well hydrated with water, and include sports drinks with 6 to 8 percent carbs if your event lasts longer than an hour.

Winning at Weight Loss

In This Chapter

- Your body's calorie-balancing act
- Why your genes may not determine your jean size
- Choosing nutrient density over energy density
- Managing your weight by listening to your body

Currently, 34 percent of Americans are classified as obese. Another 34 percent are overweight. That means less than one third of the U.S. population is walking around at a healthy weight. Excess fat on your body puts you at risk for most chronic diseases. For the first time in history, we are overfed yet undernourished. With limitless access to food resources, we're eating too much of the wrong choices and growing larger as a consequence.

Fortunately, inherent factors of a whole-food, plant-based nutrition plan naturally aid weight-loss efforts. Mind-boggling though it is—even to scientists—you can eat enough to stay satiated as you lose pounds and maintain that loss with ease.

What Counts About Calories

According to the first law of thermodynamics, energy is neither created nor destroyed, only transformed. To apply this law to your body, think of energy in terms of all the food you consume, along with how your body utilizes that food when it's absorbed. Your brain knows how much energy you require to perform all the necessary functions of daily living. When you exercise more, your appetite regulation system perks up and releases the appropriate hormones to tell you to eat more. When you're more sedentary, the opposite effect happens.

MIXED GREENS

Technically, a calorie is defined as a unit of heat required to raise the temperature of 1 kilogram of water by 1 degree at 1 atmospheric pressure. Food is measured in this way to determine how many calories are available from that item.

Your body loves to be in the state of homeostasis, or equilibrium, so it's constantly trying to balance calories to maintain a steady weight. This explains why it's challenging to lose or gain weight when your body has been stable at a set point for a while.

Theoretically, then, total calories *in* have to be less than calories *out* in order to lose weight. To maintain weight, continue to eat and burn the same amount of energy as you're currently burning. To lose, eat less and exercise more.

However, your body is a living, breathing organism that processes food through a highly complex series of reactions, and certain factors complicate the physics of calorie consumption. Not all foods are treated equally when it comes to digestion and absorption of calories. The fabulous news is that whole-plant foods complement these factors and make it easy to whittle away pounds with ease.

Genetics and Upbringing

Which came first—the chicken or the egg? Similarly, is your weight status innate or learned? The truth may lie somewhere in the middle. You may have genetic tendencies predicting how much you will weigh. Behavior patterns you learned from your family as you grew up also play a part. Which has more influence over your eating and weight tendencies? No clear-cut answer can be given yet.

Some scientists argue that genetics predict everything about your health—which diseases you're at risk for, your tendency toward obesity, how tall you'll be, and factors such as dental health and hair growth patterns. On the contrary, significant evidence suggests that genetics play a minimal role in whether these factors come to fruition.

For example, researchers at Oxford University determined in 1981 that only 2 or 3 percent of cancer risk can be attributed to genes. Furthermore, children born into poverty are thought to never reach their genetic height potential due to malnutrition. Migrant studies show clearly that incidence of obesity and chronic disease change when a person moves from one society to another. Girls are starting puberty at a younger age than their mothers did. All these findings help disprove the idea that your genetic tendencies are set in stone, unaffected by lifestyle choices.

There's plenty of room for debate. If behavior trumping genetics is correct, this unleashes the chain tying you to a variable you have zero control over—the genes you're born with. Thus, even if your DNA is set to bring on heart disease at the age of 45, you can offset that by eating a whole-food, plant-based diet; staying lean; and maintaining a consistent exercise routine.

Regardless of whether scientists agree, the take-home message is simple: you can, at the very least, set the stage for optimum health by managing your behaviors and lifestyle. Only positive benefits can come from making healthful choices. If you don't provide the fuel to the genetic fire (eating animal and processed foods, for example), lifestyle may just win over. You have absolutely nothing to lose.

Many people use their genes as an excuse to remain overweight. They give up any effort to lose weight by deciding they have no control anyway, so what's the point? Yet it's well established that overweight parents can have lean, healthy kids, and vice versa. It's time we let go of this myth that's holding back 68 percent of the U.S. population from reaching and maintaining a healthy weight. Now is the time to take back control of your body.

Phyto Factors

Whole-plant foods are ideal for weight loss. Naturally nutrient dense, plant foods are high in fiber and water content. They also contain the perfect macronutrient profile: high carbs, low to moderate protein, and low fat (except nuts, seeds, avocados, and olives).

You read about nutrient density, the level of nutrients per calorie, in Chapter 6. *Energy density* describes how many calories a food provides. To lose weight, you need to maximize your selection of nutrient-dense foods and minimize those that are energy dense.

DEFINITION

Energy density is the number of calories per gram of food (kcal/g).

Vegetables, fruits, whole grains, and legumes are high in fiber, water, vitamins, minerals, phytochemicals, and antioxidants yet low in energy density. They give the most nutritional bang for your energy buck. Foods highest in energy density also happen to be lowest in nutrient density. They include animal products, oils, and processed foods.

Eat Fiber, Lose Weight

As you learned in Chapter 4, fiber is a dietary component that passes through your stomach and small intestine without being affected by digestive processes. Many different physiological effects of fiber influence weight management.

High-fiber foods require more chewing, which may slow the rate of eating. In the stomach, fiber promotes the feeling of fullness by causing *gastric distention*. Fiber traps nutrients and slows their travel time from the stomach into the small intestine, thereby decreasing the rate of digestion. Once in the small intestine, fiber delays the absorption of nutrients and blunts the insulin rush. Some fibers (especially the ones from fruits and vegetables) even reduce the absorption of protein and fat. Thus, fiber contributes to long-term weight management throughout the course of digestion.

Together, fiber and water make up bulk, which enhances *satiety*. Increased satiety makes you feel like you've had enough to eat, contentedly allowing you to put down your fork. How many times have you eaten at a restaurant where you consumed large amounts of bread before your meal came and, somehow, you were still able to eat all your food? The bread typically served at restaurants contains little or no fiber. White bread is energy-dense and nutrient-poor—a perfect example of empty calories. If you choose fiber- and water-rich soup or a dinner salad instead of the bread as a starter, you'll be fuller and eat less of your entrée.

> **DEFINITION**
>
> **Gastric distention** is a swelling or bloating of the stomach. **Satiety** is the state of fullness and satisfaction after eating adequately.

Uncertainty among weight-loss experts is evident. Trends ebb and flow, leading optimistic dieters on one tangent and then back in the opposite direction in pursuit of the next miracle. Regardless, the one constantly accepted detail is that consuming fiber helps more than any other factor when it comes to losing weight. Focus on fiber from whole-plant foods, and you can safely and healthfully attain your goals. Fiber will never let you down, and it will help you reach and maintain your ideal body weight with ease.

Trimming the Fat

A vast amount of research shows that a diet low in fat naturally leads to weight loss when compared to higher fat intakes. A gram of fat provides 9 calories versus 4 for a gram of carbohydrate or protein. If you eat food with a higher fat percentage, you automatically consume more calories.

Interestingly, if you're eating whole-plant food sources that are higher in fat (nuts, seeds, avocados, and olives), you're also getting fiber (bonus!) and no cholesterol (another bonus!). Higher intakes of fat from processed and animal products are what promote weight gain, according to research studies. Remember that you need some fat in your diet, but too much of it will end up being stored as body fat.

To meet your daily essential fatty acid requirement, you need only the equivalent of $1\frac{1}{2}$ tablespoons ground flaxseeds, hempseeds, or chia seeds, or $\frac{1}{4}$ cup walnuts. You can also eat soybeans or leafy green veggies for these fats with a smaller caloric investment. So if your goal is to lose weight, limit your intake of high-fat foods to just the amount necessary, and don't go overboard.

Undoing the Diet Mentality

Diet books, diet plans, diet pills, and diet centers abound! If these are so readily available, why is weight loss such an obstacle? It's because quick fixes don't work. Eating for health, however, does work. It provides a long-term, easily sustainable solution. When you establish your whole-plant food eating routine, you'll lose weight, feel fabulous, and never look back.

Typical diets offer short-term plans that have you cutting out entire food groups, minimizing calories so much that you're constantly hungry, or eating a mono-diet consisting of very few choices. Of course, you can't stick with a plan like this. Who wants to suffer, starve, and not enjoy their food? You may lose weight, but the second you can't take it anymore, you'll cry mercy and go back to eating what you were before the diet … only this time with a vengeance!

This is the infamous vicious cycle known as dieting. You start a plan, lose weight, end the diet, and gain back all the weight you lost—and more! Fewer than 5 percent of dieters are able to sustain their weight loss for more than 5 years! And that's not to mention the fact that losing and gaining weight is more harmful to your health than maintaining a higher but stable weight.

Keeping It Simple

Let me introduce you to the dream diet for the new millennium. This is a life plan not only to help you lose weight, but also to achieve optimum health at the same time. Here's the simple list of recommendations to lose weight and keep it off:

- Eat only when you're truly hungry.
- Choose from any variety of whole-plant foods.
- Stop eating when you reach the feeling of satiety.
- Repeat.
- Exercise and move your body throughout the day.

That's it. Simple. Sustainable. Successful.

HEALTHY HINT

If you're not positive you're hungry, you aren't hungry. Have a cup of tea instead.

Tricks of the Trade

Previous misconceptions about dieting clog your mind, preventing you from listening to internal signals. After years of training yourself to ignore these signs, you need to relearn to notice them.

Further complicating your initial change to a diet based in whole-plant foods is your body's response; it may be trying to rid itself of the years' worth of toxins you provided. You need to understand what true hunger feels like and distinguish it from the feelings of detoxification (the process of cleansing and removing toxic compounds that may have accumulated in the organs over a period of time). Certain tricks can help you tune in to true hunger and satiety signals:

- Notice how you feel before you start eating. Ask yourself if you really *need* to eat.
- Eat only if you're hungry enough to eat an apple and all your options sound delicious.
- Pay attention to your body as you eat. Chew your food slowly, don't allow distractions while you eat (watching television, driving, etc.), and put down the fork between bites to take time to savor each bite.

- Feel your belly start to fill up, and know when you've had enough.

- When you're not hungry, don't opt to have dessert just because it's available. Either eat less of your meal to save room, or save the dessert for later when you are hungry.

If you've been a dedicated whole-food herbivore eating as recommended in this book, you should have no problem losing weight. If you notice you're plateauing or seem to be stuck, here are some tips to take it to the next level:

- Be sure you're minimizing your intake of fats.

- Avoid concentrated sweets like pure juices and dried fruits.

- Stop eating at an early hour, allowing a few hours to digest before bed. This also provides your body with a mini-fast, which offers your cells more time to repair, rebuild, and revitalize. You'll sleep better, wake up more refreshed, and be ready to break your fast with a healthy, whole-food breakfast.

- If you're starving later in the evening, closer to bedtime, eat something light, like a piece of fruit or air-popped popcorn. Forcing your body to digest something heavy while you're sleeping cuts into all the other important jobs your body needs to do during that time.

- First thing in the morning, wait until your hunger signals are obvious. Ignore all the old advice about eating at certain hours of the day, fueling your furnace, etc. Eat only when *your* body needs to eat.

- Intensify your exercise program by adding longer or more frequent sessions and increasing the challenge of each workout.

HEALTHY HINT

The more muscle tissue you have, the more calories your body requires to maintain it. Build lean muscle mass with consistent exercise.

Your body is constantly in flux, striving for homeostasis, or equilibrium. After assaults with diets and poor food choices, you may have lost touch with your intuition and actual needs. Fortunately, it's never too late to regain control. Tune in to your internal signals. Trust your body; it knows what it needs. If you emphasize delivering nutrients to your cells and ridding yourself of addictive, health-damaging compounds, your body can think clearly and shed excess weight. The same foods that promote optimum health naturally allow your body to reach its desirable size. Think simply, effortlessly, and healthfully, and you'll achieve your goals.

The Least You Need to Know

- Calories do count to a certain extent, and a whole-food, plant-based diet naturally provides low-calorie nutrient density for optimal weight management.
- Consuming fiber is the single factor experts agree on that helps promote weight loss.
- Eating foods lower in fat helps minimize caloric intake.
- Practice reconnecting your mind to your body's hunger and satiety signals. The more carefully you listen, the more natural it will become.
- For long-term weight management, eat only when you're hungry, choose whole-plant foods, and stop eating before you're full.

Dodging Disease with Diet

In This Chapter

- Overfed, undernourished, and chronically ill
- Your GI tract: gateway to good health
- Nutritional implications of common illnesses

Health-care costs are rising in harmony with disease incidence rates. Billions of dollars are being poured into new therapies, medications, procedures, and more while the patients for whom these therapies are intended grow sicker and sicker. Evidently, a key element is missing. That element is our food.

Awareness of whole-food, plant-based nutrition as an inexpensive, pain-free, and effective alternative is growing rapidly. It's been hypothesized that nutrition—as a form of prevention and treatment—can cut health-care costs by as much as 90 percent. Because researchers and health-care practitioners are seeing great successes, we're at the tipping point where food is making a comeback as "thy medicine."

Eradicating Chronic Disease

Chronic disease is considered an incurable illness. Medically speaking, for physicians treating chronic disease, the goal is symptom management, accomplished by balancing and modifying medications and offering procedures when appropriate.

According to the Centers for Disease Control, chronic diseases such as diabetes, cardiovascular disease, and cancer are the most common, costly, and preventable of all health problems in the United States. However, each of these conditions can be prevented—and many of them completely reversed—simply by adjusting lifestyle. Remember, genetics may load the gun, but lifestyle pulls the trigger.

Diabetes

Approximately 24 million Americans have diagnosed diabetes, and this number increases daily. Moreover, millions more have prediabetes. The two types of diabetes—type 1 and type 2—are different in terms of origin and mechanism.

Type 1 diabetes is an autoimmune disease—meaning it's caused by the body attacking itself—that typically begins during childhood when the pancreas is unable to produce insulin.

Type 2 diabetes occurs when the cells become resistant to insulin. In the past, type 2 diabetes was considered an adult-onset disease, but nowadays, it's being diagnosed at progressively younger ages. With both types of diabetes, blood sugar (a.k.a. blood glucose) cannot be effectively absorbed into the cells because that's the primary function of insulin. Having high levels of sugar in the bloodstream leads to major short- and long-term health consequences.

Immediate health complications of diabetes include the following:

- Diabetic ketoacidosis, a life-threatening situation caused from insufficient insulin, leading to high blood sugar levels, nausea, vomiting, abdominal pain, dehydration, ketones in the urine, acidosis, and the potential for coma and death

- Increased incidence of infections

- Insulin shock, or when too much insulin is in the blood, leading to severely low blood sugar (hypoglycemia) and possibly resulting in convulsions and coma

- Coma

- Death

Diabetes is the number-one cause of amputations and blindness. Additional long-term outcomes of diabetes include the following:

- Kidney disease

- Cardiovascular disease

- Retinopathy, a disease of the small blood vessels in the retina of the eyes that can eventually result in impaired vision and blindness

- Skin infections

- Neuropathy, or damage to the nerves that causes tingling, weakness, pain, and/or numbness usually in the legs, feet, toes, arms, and fingers

- Foot ulcers

Type 2 diabetes can be prevented, and even reversed, with diet and exercise. Obesity is the most common factor predisposing someone to type 2 diabetes, so weight management is a crucial issue. High levels of body fat lead to insulin resistance and progressively increase the need for more insulin. Eventually, this exhausts the pancreas, resulting in decreased secretion of insulin. Losing weight and exercising improve insulin sensitivity, thereby minimizing the amount of insulin necessary.

Although type 1 diabetes is an autoimmune disease, some studies have found that insulin dosing can be decreased and long-term health outcomes can be controlled with a whole-food, plant-based diet.

PLANT PITFALL

A link between early consumption of dairy and type 1 diabetes is well documented. Protein fragments from cow's milk may be absorbed into an infant's bloodstream through holes in a not yet fully developed GI tract. The immune system attacks these fragments as foreign invaders. Unfortunately, some of these proteins look like cells of the pancreas, and the body loses its ability to discern between the two types of cells. Thus, the immune system mistakenly destroys pancreatic cells as well, leading to its inability to function and produce insulin. Eventually, this process leads to type 1 diabetes, a debilitating and life-altering disease.

Around the globe, the prevalence of diabetes increases in populations that consume more saturated fat, animal fat, and animal protein. On the contrary, prevalence decreases with greater intakes of fiber and vegetable fat. Studies show an increased risk for diabetes with meat intake and with higher blood cholesterol levels. Careful control of blood sugar levels over the long haul reduces the risk of several of the complications of diabetes.

Dietary recommendations for people with diabetes used to focus on minimizing intake of carbohydrates, causing the diet to be shifted toward more protein and fat. Currently, this advice is changing due to accumulating evidence of the harm of high intakes of saturated fat and animal protein. Nutrition plans are more individualized now, and success in using whole-food, plant-based diets to reverse diabetes has been incredibly promising.

Heart Disease

Heart disease, or coronary heart disease (CHD), is the number-one cause of death in America. In most cases, heart attacks are due to a narrowing of the coronary arteries, the blood vessels that supply the heart with oxygen and nutrients. *Atherosclerotic plaque* accumulates over many years, even starting in childhood for some people, and causes this narrowing. Dr. Caldwell Esselstyn perfectly describes heart disease as a "toothless paper tiger that need never exist … and when it does exist, it need never progress."

DEFINITION

Atherosclerotic plaque is a build-up of cholesterol, calcium, cellular debris, and fatty materials in the walls of the blood vessels as a consequence of atherosclerosis.

Heart disease is essentially a food-borne illness, brought about by the overconsumption of saturated and trans fats, animal protein, and highly processed foods and the underconsumption of whole-plant foods. Coronary artery disease—the condition resulting from atherosclerosis in the arteries—is virtually nonexistent in plant-based cultures around the world.

Therapy options for heart disease—drugs, stents, and bypasses—offer no more than a band-aid effect. Truly treating the disease requires the cessation of consistently applying the source. If a sink is overflowing with water, mopping up the mess on the floor isn't going to stop the problem. That's precisely what current medical treatment does for heart disease—it mops up the water. Eating a whole-food, plant-based diet along with exercising is the equivalent of turning off the faucet.

Cancer

Cancer is the second-leading cause of death in the United States. Almost 563,000 people die from the disease every year. As poorly understood as the development and spread of cancer is, it's rather simple on the surface.

Cancer is uncontrolled, abnormal cell growth. Your cells are changing every second, constantly regenerating. On average, a healthy body produces one cancer cell a day. This leaves limitless opportunities for that one cell to go awry, leading to cancer growth. What prevents that from happening most of the time? Your immune system. If you provide your immune system with all it needs to be on its "A" game, you'll be able to fight off that abnormal cell, never knowing it was there. Feed your immune system with nutrient-dense whole foods and regular exercise to win this constant battle.

The treatments for cancer are usually worse than the cancer itself. And once again, the symptoms are targeted instead of the disease. Having to choose among amputating parts of your body, flooding your system with powerful toxins, radiating your cells, or all of the above is the worst decision you could ever have to make. Even more tragic is the fact that these treatments don't always work. Aimed at stopping the progression of the cancer, these options are simply intended to buy you time.

> **PLANT PITFALL**
>
> Certain cancers do respond well to treatment. Therapies used to treat childhood leukemia, Hodgkin's lymphoma, and germ cell tumors (as in some testicular and ovarian cancers) are typically successful. When breast and colon cancers are caught early enough, patients can have a good prognosis with treatment.

If you look at the evidence, most cancers respond extremely well to nutrition therapy—no matter how far along into the disease you happen to be. Plant-based diets have been successfully used for decades to stop cancer. The best part is, you have absolutely nothing to lose by using food. It's inexpensive, painless, delicious, and more effective than any other method.

Hypertension

Approximately one third of the U.S. population has diagnosed hypertension, or high blood pressure. Defined as a blood pressure greater than 140/90 mmHg, this condition is a primary risk factor for heart disease and stroke. Hypertension is also both a cause and a result of kidney disease.

Diet and lifestyle have been consistently found to contribute significantly to elevated blood pressure. Plant-based eaters have lower blood pressure and lower incidence of hypertension than non-plant-based eaters.

Reducing sodium intake has long been promoted as a treatment for people with hypertension. However, this conventional wisdom is controversial. For salt-sensitive individuals, this dietary adjustment may certainly be beneficial. For optimal efficacy, treatment emphasis should be on weight management; eating a whole-food, plant-based diet; and exercise.

High Cholesterol

Another primary risk factor for heart disease (and perhaps all chronic disease) is a high cholesterol level. One in every six U.S. adults has high cholesterol. The American Heart Association recommends maintaining a blood cholesterol level of less than 200 mg/dL, but the research shows that heart attacks don't occur in people with a total cholesterol level of under 150 mg/dL. Ideally, your LDL (low-density lipoprotein) should be less than 100 mg/dL, and your HDL (high-density lipoprotein) should be above 45 mg/dL.

> **MIXED GREENS**
>
> It's important to note that with a lowering of total cholesterol, HDL, the "good" cholesterol, commonly decreases, too. The role of HDL is to remove cholesterol from the blood. With less cholesterol to be removed, the need for HDL is naturally lessened. Although lower HDL levels are typically seen in plant-based populations, this is accompanied by a decreased incidence of coronary heart disease.

Cholesterol-lowering medications, especially statins, are among the most widely used drugs. Although they do what they intend (lower blood cholesterol levels), they fail to address the source of the high cholesterol. Worse, they can be toxic to the liver. No medication comes without side effects. Always opt for the drug-free path, if possible.

Cholesterol levels respond rather rapidly to diet change. Within 3 weeks of following a whole-food, plant-based plan, especially one with plenty of fiber, your cholesterol profile can take a dramatic turn for the better. Fiber acts like a sponge in your body. It soaks up cholesterol and accompanies it out of your body.

Osteoporosis

Bone is living, dynamic tissue made up of protein embedded with minerals. Calcium is the most abundant mineral found in bone, but phosphorus, magnesium, sodium, potassium, fluoride, chloride, and sulfite are also present.

Bone strength is determined by bone mineral density (BMD), or the amount of minerals in any volume of bone. After age 25 to 30, bone minerals naturally start to break down. When this process appears to be accelerated, one of two diagnoses is made, osteopenia or osteoporosis. Osteopenia is a condition in which BMD appears to be lower than normal and is considered a precursor to osteoporosis. Osteoporosis is a crippling disease that increases your risk of bone fractures. Pain, disability, diminished quality of life, and—with hip fractures—increased risk of mortality are all potential complications of osteoporosis. The disease is most common in post-menopausal women. Clinically diagnosed osteoporosis is similar between strict herbivores and omnivores; abstaining from animal products doesn't increase risk.

Claims of osteoporosis becoming epidemic have made headline news recently. Bone-building medications are flying off the physician's prescription pads as quickly as milk off the supermarket shelves. However, several caveats are evident. For the pharmaceutical, medical, supplement, and food industries, tremendous financial opportunities can be gained with medical tests, medications, supplements, and dairy products. More people with diagnosed osteoporosis equal more money to be made.

Ironically, the medications used to treat osteoporosis are not as effective as the drug manufacturers lead you to believe. Some have even been found to be dangerous. Reports have surfaced of these drugs causing esophageal cancer, heart damage, muscle pain, and other complications.

Many factors are at play when it comes to optimizing bone health, as described in Chapter 7. For prevention and reversal of osteoporosis, emphasize …

- Daily exercise, especially resistance-based exercise.

- Plenty of sunshine and possibly vitamin D supplements, if you're deficient.

- Foods rich in calcium; vegetable protein; vitamins K, C, and B_{12}; isoflavones; phytoestrogens; and omega-3 fatty acids.

Gastrointestinal Illnesses

What you put into your body via your gastrointestinal (GI) tract is your inside's link to the outside world. Your GI tract acts as a filter, deciding what may pass into the bloodstream and what has to keep on traveling back out. Hence, your immune system is greatly determined by your gut health. Ultimately, every bite determines your overall well-being. A nutrient-deficient diet plus an influx of antinutrients virtually destroys your body, beginning in your mouth.

MIXED GREENS

An entire scientific movement is in swing discovering the power of the micro-organisms that inhabit your gut. Approximately 10 trillion bacteria live in your lower gut, where they metabolize indigestible compounds and defend against harmful microbes, among other jobs. Because of the powerful interplay of immunity and your GI system, microbial ecology may be the future of medicine.

Chronic GI disorders are more prevalent than ever, and people suffer needlessly because of them. It's time to address these overly common problems by looking at the obvious—what's on your plate.

Gastroesophageal Reflux Disease

Gastroesophageal reflux disease (GERD), also known simply as reflux or heartburn, is a chronic condition caused by the regurgitation of stomach acid back up into the esophagus. Not only is GERD painful, but it can also lead to serious complications such as inflammation, ulcers, or cancer in the esophagus.

Antacids, commonly used to treat symptoms of GERD, contain high levels of aluminum, which are toxic to the brain and contribute to dementia and Alzheimer's disease. Instead of popping pills, modify your diet to avoid GERD. Behaviors that can alleviate GERD include eating a high-fiber, low-fat diet; avoiding eating past the point of comfortably full; eliminating spicy foods; sitting upright for a few hours after eating to allow the food to digest; and raising the head of your bed by 4 to 6 inches.

Inflammatory Bowel Disease

Inflammatory bowel disease (IBD) consists of two inflammatory conditions of the intestines: ulcerative colitis and Crohn's disease. Symptoms are similar between the two and include diarrhea, abdominal pain, cramping, bloody stools, and mucus. Meat, eggs, dairy, and alcohol exacerbate symptoms of these painful and debilitating diseases. Still, scientists haven't been able to establish either the cause or dietary management.

A higher prevalence of IBD is found in populations that eat meat-rich, highly processed, Westernized diets. Foods considered irritating to IBD sufferers vary, but certain ones such as alcohol, caffeine, soft drinks, wheat, sugar, high-fat foods, and yeast are common. Because of the minimized nutrient absorption found in IBD, especially during flare-ups, a nutrient-dense, plant-based diet is critical to ensure adequate intakes.

Additionally, a probiotics regimen may help support a healthy colon. Plant sources of probiotics—naturally occurring live microorganisms known to help balance the microflora in your colon—include miso, tempeh, sauerkraut, and plant-based yogurts. They are also available in supplement form.

Irritable Bowel Syndrome

Approximately 20 percent of adults suffer from irritable bowel syndrome (IBS), a chronic condition characterized by abdominal pain, cramping, bloating, and constipation and/or diarrhea. The cause of IBS perplexes health-care professionals, and it has been attributed to depression, bacterial infection, immune insufficiency, food intolerances, and stress. For some, IBS is debilitating, drastically impacting daily life.

Although medications are regularly included in treatment protocol, they're usually ineffective and, as usual, address the symptoms and not the cause. Trying to manage this disease with a high-fiber, low-fat diet along with adequate fluids may prove more beneficial. Adding foods like flaxseeds and probiotics may also improve symptoms.

Often, people suffering with IBS may have unknown food intolerances or allergies. Wheat is a common irritant, and eliminating it might help. Ask your physician to be tested for possible intolerances or allergies if you've been struggling with IBS symptoms.

Diverticular Disease

Considered a fiber-deficiency disease, diverticular disease is characterized by out-pouching and inflammation of the intestinal wall. Fiber increases stool bulk, thereby aiding its passage through the colon.

Higher fiber intake is one reason plant-based eaters enjoy a much lower incidence of this condition. High-fiber, low-fat diets in addition to exercise prevent diverticular disease.

Celiac Sprue

Celiac sprue, also known as celiac disease and gluten-sensitive enteropathy, is an auto-immune chronic disease of the digestive tract that interferes with the digestion and absorption of nutrients from food. One in 133 U.S. citizens has been diagnosed with the condition. Possibly many more cases go undiagnosed because of misdiagnosis and symptoms similar to those of food intolerances and allergies. People with celiac sprue can't tolerate gluten, a protein found in barley, rye, oats, and wheat. When consumed, celiac sufferers endure damage to the *villi* that line the intestinal tract, enabling nutrient absorption. Major concerns with celiac sprue include malnutrition and the onset of other diseases such as lymphoma, other cancers, type 1 diabetes, liver disease, lupus, rheumatoid arthritis, and thyroiditis.

Eliminating all foods and products containing gluten is the only treatment option. With a bit of information and some practice, avoiding gluten will become second nature, and a well-balanced diet is easily attained. In recent years, a whole market-place has opened for gluten-free living. Labeling of gluten has become mandatory, and thousands of alternatives to gluten are widely available. Entire stores dedicated to gluten-free shopping and restaurants with gluten-free menus are spreading rapidly.

Ingredients with gluten include wheat and wheat products (bran, bread, bread prod-ucts, wheat germ, wheat meal, wheat pasta, wheat starch, white flour, durum, wheat berries, red wheat flakes, starch, vital wheat gluten, seitan, modified food starch, modified starch, bread flour, semolina, farina, shredded wheat, wheat protein powder, cake flour); bulgur; triticale; rye; texturized vegetable protein; texturized soy protein; hydrolyzed vegetable protein; kamut; spelt; oats; barley; couscous; graham flour and graham crackers; vegetable gum; gelatinized starch; and beers, ales, and malted drinks. Look on food labels for "contains wheat" or "gluten-free" to be certain.

Carefully watching your diet is critical with celiac sprue because of the serious health complications associated with continued villi destruction.

Other Conditions

Several other chronic medical conditions have increasingly become commonplace. As poor diets become more prevalent, resultant disease ensues. Preventing and treating the following illnesses with proper nutrition have shown astonishing promise and success.

Autoimmune Disease

Your immune system is a collection of powerful tools designed to resist the constant onslaught of foreign invaders, including bacteria, viruses, and parasites. In tens of millions of Americans (75 percent of whom are women), the immune system goes awry and begins attacking itself. More than 80 diseases can be classified as autoim-mune, including multiple sclerosis (MS), rheumatoid arthritis (RA), systemic lupus erythematosus (SLE), scleroderma, type 1 diabetes, and inflammatory bowel disease (IBD; discussed earlier in this chapter). Each condition bears its own unique set of symptoms and progression of those symptoms, some localized to one body part and others systemic.

Treatment goals are to manage symptoms, delay progression, and maintain the body's ability to fight disease. Some situations call for immunosuppressants, drugs that slow immune function and increase risk of other infections.

Certain dietary interventions have shown success in reducing inflammation and medication requirements. A strict nutrient-dense diet omitting all animal products and processed foods has been found to be effective. Hidden food intolerances or sensitivities may exist, and therefore need to be assessed so they can be eliminated. Vitamin D has been implicated in autoimmune disease, especially MS, so maintain optimal blood levels of D.

Earlier in the disease process is the time to be aggressive with your diet because once the disease progresses, whatever function has been lost cannot be reversed.

Kidney Disease

An estimated 13 percent of U.S. adults suffer with chronic kidney disease (CKD). More than half a million people are treated for end-stage renal disease (ESRD), an illness in which the kidneys are unable to function adequately and require dialysis and/or a transplant.

The variety of pathology—or diseases—that occurs in the kidneys is vast and can be brought about in many different ways. The two leading causes of CKD in the United States are diabetes and high blood pressure. Other common causes include various types of chronic excessive protein intake (especially animal protein), toxicity from medications (like over-the-counter pain relievers), and *metabolic syndrome*.

Plant-based diets may help prevent and manage CKD. Both the amount and type of protein consumed impact your kidneys. High protein intake (especially from animal protein) increases *glomerular filtration rate (GFR)*. Essentially, an increased GFR means more work for your kidneys. Herbivores also have lower blood pressure and cholesterol levels, factors known to contribute to CKD incidence and progression when high.

DEFINITION

Metabolic syndrome is a cluster of conditions, including obesity, high cholesterol, hypertension, and high blood sugar, that lead to vascular and other chronic diseases. **Glomerular filtration rate (GFR)**, used to measure kidney function, is the rate at which fluid filters through the kidneys.

Dementia and Alzheimer's Disease

Dementia and Alzheimer's disease are progressive diseases of the brain that are still not clearly understood. Fortunately, you have more control over the prevention and management of both diseases than you may think.

Alzheimer's disease is the most common cause of dementia and is diagnosed specifically by the presence of senile plaques, beta-amyloid tangles, and neurofibrillary tangles inside the brain.

Treat your blood vessels well to avoid dementia and Alzheimer's disease as well as heart disease, stroke, and even erectile dysfunction. Your cardiovascular system is made up of arteries, veins, and capillaries, with your heart as the pump. These blood vessels supply nutrients and oxygen throughout your entire body, from the top of your head to the tips of your toes. Atherosclerosis, the hardening of arteries, can and does occur in any of the blood vessels. Furthermore, a high cholesterol level lends itself to all the aforementioned chronic diseases.

Dementia is a chronic deterioration of cognition that usually affects the elderly. Many varied causes are attributed, including Alzheimer's disease, vascular disease (atherosclerosis, stroke), infections, structural brain disorders (like tumors or bleeding), depression, and drugs. The progression of dementia varies according to the person, and the severity lies on a continuum. Signs of dementia include short-term memory loss; impaired ability to plan, organize, or sequence abstractly; inability to articulate ideas; and inability to make purposeful movements.

High blood cholesterol levels and atherosclerosis increase your risk of developing dementia and Alzheimer's disease. Thereby, these conditions are more prevalent in populations that eat a diet high in fat, dairy, and meat than in those following a plant-based diet. Consuming a diet rich in phytonutrients and antioxidants reduces your risk.

PLANT PITFALL

Aluminum, found in foods, cookware, water, medications (especially antacids), cans, and the air, is toxic to the nervous system and contributes to the development of dementia and Alzheimer's disease. Avoid aluminum by using non-aluminum cookware and by eliminating antacids, other aluminum-containing medications, antiperspirants, soda cans, and foods with added aluminum (like baking powder).

Gout

A painful inflammatory disease, gout results in uric acid crystal formation in the joints, usually the toes. Uric acid is a breakdown product of purines, a class of aromatic organic compounds that are components of nucleic acids (DNA and RNA) found in human and animal tissue.

Restricting foods high in purines, as well as alcohol, is recommended to alleviate symptoms of gout. Food sources high in purines include seafood, fish, organ meats (liver, kidney, heart, and sweetbreads), all other meats, and some legumes.

By now, you probably notice a trend. Diet plays a huge role in most illnesses common in the Western world. Eating a whole-food, plant-based diet prevents and reverses most of these conditions, enabling you to enjoy the freedom associated with true health.

The Least You Need to Know

- Chronic diseases like diabetes, heart disease, osteoporosis, and cancer can be prevented and even reversed by lifestyle modification.
- High blood pressure and high cholesterol are two risk factors for heart disease that are controllable with diet.
- Exercising consistently is the most important action you can take to protect your bones from osteoporosis.
- A vast majority of illnesses can be prevented and will respond favorably by eating a diet high in phytochemicals, fiber, antioxidants, vitamins, and minerals.

The Plant-Based Recipe Box

Now that you know why whole-food, plant-based nutrition can rock your world in the best way possible, it's time to get cooking and eating! In Part 4, I share strategies to help you maintain an environment in which health-promoting foods are constantly available.

Being an herbivore need not turn you into a recluse. Dining out is easy if you know what to look for, as is attending social gatherings. In Chapter 17, I fill in all the odds and ends on how to master these techniques.

And for all the times you're happily at home, Chapters 18 and 19 give you a simple formula so that you're ready to cook at the first strike of hunger. You learn how to stock your kitchen and substitute ingredients so you can always have delicious plant fare at your fingertips. I also show you how to nutrify your favorite recipes, and I share some new ones—more than 45 in all!—to add to your collection. Being prepared is the key to long-term triumph.

Àvotre santé! To your health!

Plant-Based in the Real World

In This Chapter

- An ounce of preparation is worth a pound of hunger
- Plant-based dining out and about
- Wholesome holiday eating
- Plant-based entertaining

After learning all about plant-based nutrition in the preceding chapters, your curiosity and enthusiasm must be bursting at the seams! Ready to take it on-the-go?

While the rest of the world rapidly catches up as the buzz progressively grows louder, you'll still find a few challenges to contend with when eating away from home. Regardless, a little careful thought goes a long way and helps sustain you on your path of plant-based bliss.

Lessons in Preparation

In life, luck happens when opportunity meets preparation. No matter the goal, you should always be prepared to face obstacles. A little homework and planning make every situation flow smoothly.

At home, you can easily arrange to have a plethora of plants available to eat at all times by shopping regularly and preparing some basic items. A major benefit of eating at home is that you always know what's going into your meals if you're making them yourself. The stability, flexibility, and comfort of having control are key components to maintaining ease in your eating.

However, it's not always possible, or even fun, to hang out at home all the time. Being a recluse is not a prerequisite for a healthy diet! As a matter of fact, dining out and enjoying meals at the homes of your friends and family are fantastic opportunities. Not only do you get to experience dishes created by someone besides yourself, but you also have the chance to inspire and motivate others.

So let's get packing, strategizing methods to bring the plant-based world along for the ride!

Fail to Plan, Plan to Fail

Who likes being stuck in a meaty situation where you have no options? Rather than finding yourself uncomfortably starving with no whole plants to devour, plan out every adventure. Traveling? Bring enough food with you to last until you'll be near dining options. At work all day? Pack snacks and meals or search out appropriate nearby restaurants to obtain adequate nutrition. Think like a scout, and treat every occasion as an adventure.

Planning is pleasurable because you'll derive comfort from knowing you'll have food as needed. Plus, you'll enjoy opportunities for new discoveries. Who knew a great plant-based restaurant was within walking distance from your workplace? Look at how many grab-and-eat choices are available at your local grocery store! Fine-tune your whole-plant vision, and the world will open itself to you. You need never go hungry nor feel isolated in any situation again!

Packing Meals and Snacks

When packing a to-go lunch, so many opportunities for creativity abound. You can vary your options from simple to gourmet, depending on where you're going and what you have on hand at home.

Plant foods travel exceedingly well. Some, in fact, are born ready to go straight from nature. Whole fruits are nature's portable candy—just rinse and enjoy anywhere and anytime. Visit your local farmers' market regularly to stock up on freshly picked direct-from-the-farm produce. Raw nuts and seeds are also quick to grab and offer nutrient-dense, hunger-satiating calories.

HEALTHY HINT

In the bulk section of your supermarket, buy large bags of dried fruits, raw nuts, and raw seeds so you can whip up your own bags of trail mix. These make an easy, satisfying whole-food snack that lasts a long time, requires no refrigeration, and travels compactly.

Have you noticed the wall of nutrition bars in the market nowadays? Dozens of options line the shelves. Because of their convenience factor, nutrition bars are big sellers, and some can fit into your whole-food, plant-based diet.

When selecting a bar, be sure the ingredients list contains only whole foods. Fortunately, this requirement won't limit you much because several product lines are based on whole foods. Stock up on these, and use them as an emergency snack. They'll stay fresh for months (always read expiration dates, of course, because the more whole the product, the fewer preservatives to extend freshness), and they travel extremely well.

You can even make your own bars at home. Although they don't last as long, they're delicious, and the ingredients are 100 percent under your control. Try AJ's Peanut Bites (recipe in Chapter 23).

Leftovers can make exciting and satisfying on-the-go meals. Invest in storage containers—preferably glass or stainless steel instead of plastic or aluminum—with tight-fitting lids. Last night's dinner usually tastes better the next day after the flavors have had time to meld. Casseroles, soups, stir-fries, salads, loaves, grains, legumes, and patties all travel easily with the proper storage containers.

Sandwiches offer no limit to creativity. Using tortillas, rice wrappers, or nori sheets as wraps or sprouted, whole-grain breads for a classic sandwich, you can create masterpieces. Imaginative style options include sushi, Noritos (see recipe in Chapter 20), burritos, and traditional sandwich fashion. Add spreads like hummus, guacamole, bean dip, and nut butters, and top with sliced, chopped, or whole veggies to boost phytonutrients, textures, and flavors. Banana slices with nut butter is a delicious classic. Hummus goes gorgeously with tomatoes and cucumbers. Sprouts can be added to any spread to really kick it up a nutrient notch. Of course, glorious greens should be used at any opportunity for every nutritional benefit.

If you want to forego the sandwich, turn the spreads into dips by packing them in small containers. Bring along dippers like cut carrots, bell peppers, celery, jicama, or other veggies; corn or rice thins; or homemade pita or tortilla chips.

HEALTHY HINT

Baked potatoes—any variety, but especially sweet potatoes or yams—are decadent, nutrient-filled snacks. Bake several at a time and store them in the fridge. Grab one when you're on the way out the door, and enjoy it either cold or warmed up.

Visiting the supermarket or health food store for quicker, last-minute choices is also an option. Convenience items have grown in abundance and variety. For a few extra cents (or bucks, depending on where you buy), you can have prewashed, precut veggies; salads; and fruits. These options are perfect if you have limited prep time. (To save money, prep in advance so you can grab and pack as necessary.) Salad bars are more robust nowadays and brimming with healthful, whole-plant foods. If you're planning to travel by plane, train, or bus, bringing a huge salad will last you several hours and keep you happily crunching until you reach your destination. Include plenty of beans, lentils, grains, and seeds for more substantial sustainability.

Prepared foods are a little trickier to navigate because most recipes contain large amounts of oil, salt, and animal products. Great take-out items at your market can include freshly made sushi vegetable rolls, plain cooked grains or legumes, steamed veggies, or baked potatoes. Sauces can be a killer, so avoid them unless you happen to know every ingredient included. Look for the cleanest, most natural choices, and don't be afraid to ask questions.

Dining Out

No restaurant is impossible to navigate, even with the strictest guidelines and highest hopes for a healthful meal. Ethnic cuisine offers tremendous variety in delicious plant-based fare. Even at a steakhouse, where the options seem narrow, you can create a meal to savor.

Check Menus Ahead of Time

Do you even remember life before the Internet? Talk about the ultimate in convenience! Most restaurants now post their menus on their websites so you have access to them at any time. Homework was never this easy! If you know ahead of time which restaurant you'll be dining at, take a look at the menu before you head out so you have time to make a careful decision.

If nothing seems to meet your criteria, you can also call ahead and ask if the chef is willing to work with you. Although the answer is almost always a resounding "Of course!" if the chef is less than accommodating, maybe choose another restaurant.

MIXED GREENS

Great websites are available now to help you pinpoint the type of restaurant that will cater to your needs. See Appendix D for recommendations.

Because a surge of people have either food allergies or sensitivities, are on some sort of special "diet," or have specific preferences, most food establishments are equipped to respond to such requests.

Nutrifying Any Restaurant

You're on a mission. At whichever restaurant you choose, you need to find whole-plant foods devoid of oil and other processed foods. An efficient method of selecting your perfect order should go like this:

Scan the menu in its entirety—from appetizers through desserts—and assess the whole-ness (or lack thereof) of the menu choices. Determine what sounds good to you by silently tuning in and asking yourself what you're hungry for. In the mood for something light? Starving and need something more substantial? If your choice is already full of colors, comes packed with fiber, and meets the criteria for the whole-food, plant-based plan, you're ready to order.

Ask the waitperson if the dish can be prepared without oil and with any sauce or dressing on the side. If you plan on using them, be sure you know what's in the sauces. Most sauces and dressings have oil, dairy, and a lot of salt. Ask if a restaurant has options without these ingredients. Typically safe choices include any vinegar, mustard, fresh marinara sauce, fresh salsa, and fresh guacamole.

If no menu options pop off the page as plant-friendly, don't worry. You can mix and match to create your own meal. Glance at all the individual items throughout the menu so you become familiar with what they have in the kitchen. Then request those items as a customized entrée.

 HEALTHY HINT

Supplement whatever you order with a side salad and/or veggie side dishes. Ask for steamed veggies—or grilled, if the chef will prepare them without oil. Remember, the more color on your plate, the more blissful your cells.

Working with the Waitstaff and Chef

Most of the time, your waitperson and/or chef will be open to constructing a meal that meets your needs. Between the creativity inherent in a chef and the common endeavor for customer satisfaction, a request for something off the menu may be an inspiring challenge.

As long as you're pleasant, appreciative, and specific about what you want, a good restaurant will accommodate you as much as possible.

Finding Something at a Steakhouse

Different types of restaurants provide new prospects for whole, plant-based cuisine. Some have more options than others, but you'll almost always find enough to fill your belly.

Vegan/vegetarian, Asian, Indian, and Mexican give you almost too many choices to decide from. But even a steakhouse can have some herbaceous helpings. You can always ask your waitperson what's on the menu that's free of meat, dairy, eggs, and oil if you're not sure or you want some other ideas. Who knows? Maybe specials are unlisted or other meals don't appear on the menu.

Brilliant menus at exclusively veg establishments are on the rise. Imagine what joy you'll feel when you find an entire menu that's plant-friendly! All you need to be wary of is oil, agave, white breads, and other processed foods. Other than that, you can have a field day sampling inventive plant fare.

Traditional Asian cuisine is plant-based. In rural Asian cultures, citizens thrive on rice, vegetables, and a bit of soy for flavor. Westernized Chinese restaurants are meat-heavy but also typically offer steamed tofu, steamed vegetables, and brown rice. You can add a side salad with rice vinegar and Chinese mustard as a dressing. Beware of deep-fried dishes and rich sauces. Spring rolls with tofu and vegetables make for excellent appetizers as long as they're not fried.

Japanese food is plant-friendly, with a wide variety of foods to choose from. Veggie sushi options include avocado rolls, vegetable rolls, and cucumber rolls. Other first-class choices include sunomono (cucumber) salad; steamed, unsalted edamame (soybeans); and seaweed salad.

Many Indians traditionally maintain a vegetarian diet, so finding healthful options is easy at Indian restaurants. Additionally, Indian food is incredibly spiced, exploding with flavor and tantalizing to the taste buds. Dishes such as aloo gobi (cauliflower and potatoes), vegetable biryani, and chana masala (curried, tomato-y chickpeas) are scrumptiously satisfying. Because most Indian restaurants go heavy on the oil, ask if you can have your servings oil-free or which dishes they serve already oil-free.

Nothing says fiesta like a Mexican meal. Screaming with the colors of the Mexican flag (red, white, and green), meals are spiced with cilantro and onion and are welcoming for herbivores. Indulge with vegetable fajitas made oil-free on corn tortillas, rice and beans, salad with salsa and guacamole, or a combination wrapped up into a burrito or taco. *Muy delicioso!*

PLANT PITFALL

When eating Mexican, ask whether the beans are made with lard (animal fat) or pork, as this is common practice. Also be sure the rice isn't cooked in animal broth.

Let's not forget about that steakhouse, where one person's side dish is another person's entrée. Explore your plant options in the side dish category. Baked potatoes, steamed veggies, corn on the cob, brown rice, beans, salad, and asparagus are standard fare. Although this may not be your first choice, it's comforting to know you can find tasty whole foods to eat if the circumstances are out of your hands.

Holidays and Special Occasions

Holidays are cause for family and friends to unite, usually surrounding a shared meal. Once you adopt whole-food, plant-based eating as a way of life, you want to tailor every aspect to optimize your well-being. Fortunately, special occasions can inspire new traditions still focused around celebration while honoring your whole-food goals.

PLANT PITFALL

Get-togethers tend to bring opportunities for others who don't understand your journey to question you about your choices. Respond honestly to his or her questions, and be gentle, not preachy or judgmental. Your choices bring to light the deficits and risks of the other person's lifestyle, drawing him or her to the point of discomfort. Offer a copy of this book so he or she can explore the miraculous plant-based world!

Use the opportunity to explore inventive recipes and share your new world with the people closest to you. Win over your family and friends by introducing delectable foods. Woo them through their palates so they understand why you've easily revolutionized your diet. Show your loved ones how even a celebratory event presents no need for sacrifice. Whole-plant versions of almost every traditional dish you've known and loved your entire life are available—and, most important, scrumptious.

How to Eat on the Holidays

Food and festivities define holiday culture. Healthful habits tend to fly out the window with the onslaught of parties, stress, and an abundance of junk foods perpetually dancing their way past your eyes and nose. So what's a whole-plant foodie to do?

To maintain consistency, focus on your goals and the pleasure of your accomplishments thus far. Eating a whole-food, plant-based diet has changed your taste buds and every cell in your body. You've conquered your addictions. You may have even reversed your disease or stopped requiring medications. Using the holidays as an excuse to break your cycle of progress and achievement is counterproductive and can start a downward spiral back to your old habits. It's not worth it.

HEALTHY HINT

Allow exercise to be your rock throughout the holiday season (as well as the rest of the year). Rely on it, and it will consistently support your efforts to stay focused mentally, emotionally, and, of course, physically.

The allure and seduction of comfort foods originate from the situation in which you consumed them, not the foods themselves. You may crave pumpkin pie on Thanksgiving because you associate it with time spent with loved ones. But it's the memories that seduce your mind masked as the pumpkin pie. Now is a critical time in your life to create new associations. Start an annual before-dinner walk/run/hike on Thanksgiving morning with your family and friends. Schedule a holiday green smoothie competition, with prizes for the yummiest concoctions. Join fellow herbivores for potlucks and gatherings to celebrate birthdays and other special occasions. Create your new life, and make it joyful. Nothing in the world tastes better than excellent health feels.

To inspire you during the holidays, write down a specific set of goals to get you through the season. List your time-stamped, detailed, accountability-based goals on paper, and put that paper where you will see it at least once a day. Keep it in your pocket or purse, if you need to. Why do you need to maintain your new habits? What do you want to achieve in the next day, week, month, or year?

HEALTHY HINT

New Year's resolutions are the perfect way for you to start your year. You can also write birthday resolutions if your birthday isn't too close to January 1. Let this be your introspective source for inspiration each year. What do you want to accomplish this year?

Logistical methods can ensure plant-based holiday maintenance. You should never be in a situation where you're stuck without healthful options. Plan to succeed by thinking ahead.

When attending parties, ask the host if whole-plant options will be available, and regardless of the answer, offer to bring a dish. That way, you're guaranteed to have something you know you'll love. Most party fare includes some sort of veggies and fruit. To fill in the potential gaps, bring a hearty dish to serve as your main course. Dishes such as a lentil loaf, lasagna, or bean chili make great party favorites that will entice all the guests' curiosity. If you're extra motivated, bring a dessert as well because whole-plant desserts are hard to come by.

At work during the holidays, the unwhole and unplant foods seem relentlessly in your face. Co-workers tend to incite sugar comas and fatty-food lethargy by inundating the office with not-so-healthy treats. No wonder people are sick so often around this time of year! The old tale of cold weather causing colds and flus is inaccurate and missing a crucial link. When your diet is inadequate, your immune system is compromised.

Fill your workspace with easy-to-grab goodies to keep temptation from taking over. Be sure you pack enough food to last you all day, and include treats you love. Remind yourself that if a piece of fresh fruit doesn't sound good, you probably aren't really hungry.

If the celebratory indulgences are becoming too much, take a walk to get some fresh air; drink hot tea; or reward yourself with a mental break by calling a friend, checking your favorite website, or listening to music with your earphones.

MIXED GREENS

Your support system is critical to your long-term success. Surround yourself with people who understand your intentions and who genuinely care about your outcomes.

Finally, experimenting with new recipes is always fun around the holidays, regardless of your nutrition plan. Stay tuned for tips on converting recipes to meet your needs in Chapter 19. Preparing wholesome plant cuisine stimulates all your senses and is a relaxing, educational, and pleasurable way to connect with your loved ones.

Entertaining with Veg Style

Excuses for entertaining are infinite. Whether for a small or large gathering, a holiday party or simple get-together, or a casual or sophisticated party, feeding gracious guests can be so satisfying. Enjoying nutritiously decadent plant fare is a superb way to bond and inspire.

If your guests aren't fellow herbivores, don't pressure yourself into thinking this meal has to represent the be-all and end-all of whole-food cooking. Instead, choose your favorite dishes and/or explore new ones. You'll tantalize your visitors when you …

- Use color copiously throughout the courses. Visual appeal initiates the journey of flavor.

- Alter the textures and flavors among dishes. If each dish is similar in texture and/or flavor, it could get a little boring for your guests.

- Choose a theme to add to the festivities. Mexican Fiesta, Poetry on a Plate, Autumnal Equinox, Beach Party, High Tea, 1980s Flashback, or Breakfast-for-Dinner are some ideas to spice up and focus your party.

Regardless of the occasion, entertain effortlessly by considering the meal a chance to share information and recipes and stimulate the senses. Open minds with a warm and welcoming home.

The Least You Need to Know

- Choose your own eating adventure by planning ahead. Be certain to bring adequate healthful choices to sustain you until you'll be somewhere plentiful in plants.

- Leftovers, sandwiches, wraps, and raw fruits and vegetables travel easily with some containers and a bit of imagination.

- Wise choices make for successful dining adventures and are possible in almost any restaurant.

- Never hesitate to ask questions when ordering at a restaurant. You need to know that what you're eating fits into your whole-food eating plan.

- Focus on your long-term goals during special occasions and holidays. Support your nutrient-dense, health-promoting diet by always having optimal food choices available, planning carefully, and surrounding yourself with support.

- Feeding friends and family wholesome plant delicacies is a decadent way to bond.

The Plant-Based Kitchen

In This Chapter

- Preparing your plant-friendly kitchen
- The culinary equipment you need
- Updating to wholesome alternatives

Doesn't all this talk about wholesomely decadent plant provisions make you hungry? It's time to stock your kitchen with the staples necessary to make delicious, nutritious, plant-based meals at home.

In this chapter, I show you how to establish your new favorite foods, dishes, and tools by taking the time to try new techniques. Plus, I share tips on how you can substitute and replace some of your old ingredients—like eggs and cheese—with health-promoting versions by using a few tweaks and tricks.

Stocking Up

Certain items should always be planted in your kitchen so you have the freedom to throw a dish together at a moment's notice. Of course, shelf- or freezer-stable ingredients can be stockpiled for longer without worrying about a rapid expiration date. Produce will naturally need to be replaced more regularly.

Stocking Your Pantry

A perfect plant-based pantry is ideally stocked with a variety of longer-lasting items, including these:

- Brown rice
- Wild rice
- Oats
- Quinoa
- Amaranth
- Barley
- Buckwheat
- Wheat berries
- Bulgur
- Dried peas, lentils, and all beans
- Almond, oat, hemp, soy, and other unsweetened milks
- Canned beans (ideally salt-free and BPA-free)
- Purées like pumpkin, sweet potato, pear, and applesauce
- Canned tomatoes
- Canned tomato paste
- Canned corn
- Canned water chestnuts
- Canned artichoke hearts, packed in water
- Raw tahini
- Raw nut butters
- Olives
- Roasted red peppers, packed in water
- Dried dates
- 100 percent pure date syrup (Find it in specialty stores, or learn how to make your own in Chapter 19.)

- Hot sauces and salsas

- Balsamic, red wine, rice wine, apple cider, and other vinegars

- Blackstrap molasses

- 100 percent pure maple syrup

- Whole-grain pasta (corn, whole-wheat, brown-rice, quinoa, or soy)

- Whole-grain crackers, corn thins, and brown-rice cakes

- Whole-grain flour (oat, barley, and whole-wheat, for example)

- Dried fruits

- Sun-dried tomatoes

- Unopened raw nuts and seeds (refrigerate after opening)

- Raw cacao nibs

- Cocoa powder

To stay well supplied, maintain ongoing shopping lists. As soon as you open the last of an item from your pantry, add it to your list for the next time you go food shopping. That way, you won't forget and will always have those ingredients ready when you need them.

What's in the Fridge?

How delightful is it to open your refrigerator and see bright, colorful options, ready to be devoured whenever hunger strikes? All you need is a bit of planning and a shopping/prepping plan to keep you fully supplied. The refrigerator represents a temporary storage house where perishables move quickly and, ideally, are consumed in appropriate time.

In your fridge, store the following:

- Open plant milks, sauces, tahini, salsas, vinegars, and oil-free salad dressings

- Open flaxseeds, hempseeds, chia seeds, raw nuts, and nut butters

- Fresh veggies

- Salads

- Leftovers

- Cut fruits

- Whole-fruit jams

- Fresh dill, rosemary, basil, cilantro, parsley, and other herbs

- Tofu

- Tempeh

- Jars of minced garlic and ginger

- Whole-grain corn, brown-rice, whole-wheat, or sprouted-grain tortillas

To boost convenience and maintain an easy-grab situation to keep you on track, always keep cut veggies and fruits, a salad, a soup, and bean dip in your fridge. These foods make perfect snacks and supplements to your main dish. You can also keep batches of leftover grains or beans to toss into whatever you're preparing for dinner. Bags of prewashed leafy greens are ideal for quickly throwing together your morning green smoothie, so keep those handy, too.

Foods from the Freezer

Your freezer can be a convenient dream come true if you know how to use it the right way. Take advantage of extra time or leftovers by freezing full meals and saving them for occasions when you're too busy to cook. Make extra portions when you do have cooking opportunities or a food-prep fest, and freeze the extras in freezer-friendly storage containers. Also, sustain an adequate supply in your freezer of the following:

- Frozen bananas and other fruits (organic, if possible)

- Frozen peas, greens, broccoli, mushrooms, mixed blends, and other vegetables

- Precooked brown rice

- Whole-fruit popsicles or sorbet

HEALTHY HINT

Frozen bananas make green smoothies divine by hiding any bitterness of the greens and providing a creamy texture. Buy extra bananas every week, and when they reach the state of ripeness you prefer, peel them, break them into halves or thirds, and store them in freezer storage containers in the freezer.

Herbs and Spices

Plain salt and pepper are so ... well, plain. Today's seasoning zing originates from creative blends, fresh herbs, and organic dried spices. Why be bland when you can explode with flavor? Bring out the essence of whole-plant foods by experimenting with seasonings.

Herbs are plants valued for their aromas, flavors, or medicinal qualities. The most commonly used fresh herbs include the following:

• Basil	• Oregano
• Chives	• Parsley
• Cilantro	• Rosemary
• Dill	• Sage
• Mint	• Thyme

These herbs can be used dried as well.

Spices are any of a variety of dried seeds, roots, bars, fruits, or leaves used to add flavors, colors, or antimicrobial properties to foods. Classic dried spices commonly used include the following:

• Allspice	• Garlic powder
• Anise	• Ginger
• Cardamom	• Lemongrass
• Cayenne	• Mace
• Chili	• Marjoram
• Cinnamon	• Mustard
• Cloves	• Nutmeg
• Coriander	• Onion powder
• Cumin	• Oregano
• Curry	• Paprika
• Fennel	• Pepper

- Red pepper flakes
- Thyme
- Sage
- Turmeric
- Star anise

If you're ready to have some real fun (or you need help with being daringly flavorful), spice blends are for you. Sprinkle them on any mix of legumes, grains, and veggies to create a flavor sensation. Check the ingredient list to be sure your store-bought blends are salt-free. And always remember that less is more when experimenting. You can always add more, but you can't take it out once it's in!

The following table lists the spices used to create popular spice blends. (Note that blends vary by brand.)

Popular Spice Blends

Blend Name	Ingredients
Chili powder	Garlic powder, onion powder, ground cumin, ground oregano, ground allspice
Chinese five-spice powder	Ground star anise, ground fagara, ground cassia seeds, ground cloves, ground fennel seeds
Curry powder	Ground red chiles, ground coriander seeds, ground mustard seeds, ground black peppercorns, ground fenugreek seeds, ground ginger, ground turmeric
Garam masala	Ground cumin, ground coriander seeds, ground cardamom, ground black peppercorns, ground cloves, ground cinnamon, ground mace, ground bay leaves
Herbes de Provence	Basil, fennel, marjoram, rosemary, sage, thyme
Jerk seasoning	Minced dried chiles, ground thyme, ground cinnamon, ground ginger, ground allspice, ground cloves, minced dried garlic, minced dried onions
Pickling spice	Mustard seeds, red pepper flakes, allspice berries, dill seed, cinnamon stick, mace, whole cloves, bay leaves, dried ginger
Quatre-Épices	Grated nutmeg, ground whole cloves, ground ginger, ground black peppercorns
Zahtar	Ground sumac, roasted sesame seeds, dried thyme

Dried herbs and spices are stronger in flavor than their fresh counterparts due to a concentration of the phytochemicals in the dried form. Basically, you're getting more of the herb or spice because the water is taken out. Store dried varieties in a cool, dark, dry location to maintain freshness.

The general rule for measuring fresh versus dried herbs is that 1 tablespoon fresh is the equivalent of 1 teaspoon dried. Powdered versions are even more potent than crumbled because they disperse throughout the food more easily. You can alternate between the two based on the recipe requirements and what you have in your kitchen or garden. Fresh is ideal in terms of flavor but much less convenient than dried. Dried spices are shelf-stable for 2 or 3 years when kept in a cool, dry place in airtight containers. You can tell when a dried spice is no longer good when its aroma disappears.

MIXED GREENS

User-friendly kits to grow your own herb garden abound. You can cultivate your own herbs in your kitchen, backyard, or anywhere else you like. Whether you have a green thumb or not, fresh and fragrant herbs can be yours with ease.

New to herbs and spices and not sure what to use with what? No problem! The following table outlines some commonly recognized herbs and spices used around the world in traditional cuisine.

Spices Around the World

Region	Herbs and Spices
Asian	Cinnamon, cloves, fennel, pepper, star anise
Indian	Coriander, cumin, curry, mustard, turmeric
Italian	Basil, oregano, parsley, rosemary, thyme
Mediterranean	Cumin, garlic, onion, pepper, turmeric
Mexican	Basil, chili powder, cilantro, cumin, onion
Southwestern United States	Chili powder, garlic, onion powder, paprika
Thai	Chili, cilantro, lemongrass, Thai basil

Equipped to Veg Out

Nothing special is required to be a full-fledged whole-plant foodie. Any basically equipped kitchen is adequate to get you started. Of course, gadgets and equipment are available to do all sorts of fancy tricks and to make life easier. So you can stay basic or indulge your technical or curious side, depending on your budget and preferences.

Basic Appliances

Two of the most valuable small appliances for your kitchen are the food processor and the blender. Your food processor doesn't have to be top-of-the-line to get the job done, but having something to chop, mix, slice, grate, mince, and shred saves you time and increases your productivity.

If you can invest in one item for your kitchen, it should be a high-powered blender. This appliance is so strong, it could turn a hockey puck into liquid. Making green smoothies with one of these powerhouses is simple because nothing combines and liquefies with the same gusto.

An immersion blender is an inexpensive, super-handy tool that allows you to bring the blender to the food instead of the other way around. Ideal for puréeing hot soup right in the pan, it's easy to use and clean.

Rice/vegetable steamers are useful because they enable you to make whole grains as simply as possible. Just add the grain and the water in the appropriate ratio, and push the setting. Voilà! Within minutes, you have perfectly steamed grains without a mess, a burnt pot, or the need to stir every few minutes. Plus, the steamer keeps it warm until you're ready to serve your meal. You can also throw in your veggies at the end for an easy steam.

Slow cookers are ideal in the plant-based kitchen. Slow cookers' set-it-and-forget-it ease of use makes cooking meals effortless. If you can open ingredients, you can have delicious dishes ready to eat whenever you are.

Other equipment, like pressure cookers, juicers, dehydrators, and coffee grinders, are some beyond-the-basic small appliances that will inspire you and/or save time.

Handy Utensils

A good set of knives is crucial. Herbivores spend much time chopping away and need to maximize efficiency as much as possible. Most important are a chef's knife, a serrated bread knife, a smaller serrated knife (for cutting tomatoes), and a paring knife. Your chef's knife will become an attachment to your hand because you'll need it to chop and prep veggies frequently. Invest in one you love, and to make chopping time trouble-free, keep it sharp with an effective sharpener.

Kitchen scissors are a must-have for cutting veggies and herbs and opening bags. You may consider doubling up on the scissors, reserving one for food only to prevent cross-contamination.

You'll also need a cutting board. Bamboo is a sustainable material, it's beautiful, and it doesn't contain the harmful chemicals found in plastic. Another perk of omitting animal products is that you don't need separate cutting boards for meats and produce to prevent cross-contamination.

PLANT PITFALL

Plastics are ubiquitous, found in everything from wrappers, storage containers, and food products to baby bottles and toys. As convenient and accommodating as plastic is, it also comes with health implications. Chemicals found in plastics, such as dioxins, phthalates, and bisphenol A (BPA), are known to damage the immune system, alter hormones, and cause cancer.

Peelers, zesters, and graters are utensils mandatory for certain effects. You'll need one of each to help massage the phyto-fabulous complexes of citrus, roots, potatoes, and more.

Must-Haves and Lovely Luxuries

Pots, pans, and mixing bowls are essential in any kitchen. Depending on how many people you're cooking for and what types of recipes you typically conjure up, the sizes and shapes you need may vary. The materials these items are made from matter most. Plastics, many metals like aluminum, and the nonstick chemicals release toxins into your foods as they cook or just come into contact with these substances. Choose cast iron, stainless steel, bamboo, glass, enamel, or silicone as safe and functional options.

Measuring cups and spoons are also kitchen fundamentals. Aim for glass or stainless steel with clearly defined measurements.

You'll also need a colander, can opener, spatulas, large wooden spoons, ladle, tongs, whisk, baking sheets, and oven mitts.

Now for the "lovely luxuries." These items aren't critical but add opulence and flair. Included in this category are the wooden citrus reamer, apple corer, veggie chopper, tofu press, mandoline, spiral slicer, (plant) milk frother, garlic press, mezzaluna, melon baller, and silicone bakeware.

Plant-Based Substitutions

Afraid you'll miss your go-to favorites? Hooked on meat or cheese? Wonder how to bake without eggs? If so, check out the sparkling substitutions in the plant world. These alternatives not only taste luscious but are also healthful!

Egg Replacements

Eggs are versatile in both cooking and baking. The high protein and fat content help bind, leaven, and thicken and also increase tenderness, volume, and richness. Fortunately, you have several options when it comes to egg substitutions, depending on what type of recipe you're creating.

Commercial egg replacers, commonly found in most health food stores, are typically flavorless and can, therefore, be used in a sweet or savory dish. You must add water to these powders to create an egglike consistency. Usually the measurements are $1\frac{1}{2}$ teaspoons commercial egg replacer (like Ener-G or Bob's Red Mill) mixed with 2 tablespoons warm water for 1 egg, but follow the directions on the package for the accurate ratio.

Soft tofu works magnificently in quiches, scrambles, frittatas, or egg salads. Sometimes crumbled firmer tofu provides a more similar texture to cooked egg. Adding turmeric turns the tofu yellow and, in some dishes, might be unrecognizable to unsuspecting tasters. For a baked good, blending silken tofu with liquid ingredients until smooth doesn't change the flavor but makes the dish heavier. This technique is ideal for brownies. When making substitutions, $\frac{1}{4}$ cup blended soft tofu is the equivalent of 1 large egg.

When baking, smashed or puréed fruits work wonders. Substitute $\frac{1}{2}$ banana or $\frac{1}{4}$ cup puréed fruit like applesauce per 1 egg.

Flax "eggs" are awe-inspiring. When made correctly, they look, feel, and act exactly like egg whites, but without the health burden! Blend, mix, or whisk 1 tablespoon ground flaxseed with 3 tablespoons water until the mixture turns into a thick, white milkshake consistency. Use for dressings, sauces, mayonnaise, or baked goods.

Chia seeds have an identical effect and can be used in the same way, except the ratio is 1 teaspoon ground chia seeds to 3 tablespoons water.

MIXED GREENS

Flaxseeds and chia seeds are chock-full of omega-3 fatty acids, fiber, and other phytonutrients. Plus, the cost of making an egg substitute with these ingredients is pennies.

Plant Milks

A plethora of plant-based milks (or mylks) have flooded the marketplace in response to consumer demand. Whether for lactose intolerance or other health reasons, many people are turning to these delicious and nutritious dairy substitutes.

Each type of milk provides its unique texture and flavor, and most are fortified to the extent that nothing is lacking nutritionally when compared to the dairy version. Here are some options you might want to check out:

- Soy milk is creamy, smooth, and rich—perfect for adding to your morning coffee or tea. It is rich in nutrition and substitutes directly (with the same ratio) in all recipes.

- Rice milk is grainier and thinner and is lower in protein and other nutrients. However, rice is the least allergenic food available, so this product works well for people with allergies or who simply prefer the texture.

- Oat milk is even grainier, but it's thicker than rice milk. Plus, it provides some fabulous fiber to the mix.

- Hemp milk is a more recent addition to the club, offering some of hemp's famous omega-3 fatty acids.

Regardless of your preference, select the unsweetened version to avoid added sugars. Also, confirm that the product is fortified with vitamins B_{12} and D by reading the ingredients list.

Mock Meats

Odds are, you were raised on the standard American diet based on meat and potatoes. Meat and meat products are typically the centerpiece of the dinner plate, with a potato and maybe some veggies on the side. Because of this tradition, switching to an entirely new plate display may be difficult at first. This is where mock meats—or meat analogues intended to imitate the texture, flavor, and appearance of meats but made from non-animal-based ingredients—come into play.

Every time I visit the supermarket, it appears as though new plant-based products have popped onto the shelves. The creativity and quality of these meat-imitating items are rather impressive, making perfect transition foods or special treats.

Truth be told, these meat alternatives aren't definitive of health foods. However, the fact that they replace animal products makes them, by default, *healthier* foods. Although they're processed, mock meats are devoid of animal protein, cholesterol, and (most of the time) saturated fat. Plus, their contribution to enabling meat-eaters to go meatless offers inherent benefit.

PLANT PITFALL

Textured vegetable protein (TVP), or textured soy protein, is a highly processed meat analogue used in several vegan products. Claims that TVP contains large amounts of MSG—and possibly even aluminum—warrant further investigation before confirming the safety of its use.

Once you're past the transition states, more whole foods will naturally take precedence in your diet as your taste buds change and your plant-based recipe box grows. Ultimately, mock meats should be thought of as an occasional indulgence.

Tofu, Tempeh, and Seitan

Nutritionally, tofu is a rich source of protein, omega-3 fatty acids, calcium (if prepared with calcium sulfate), iron, and isoflavones. Tofu comes in a range of firmnesses, from soft to extra-firm. Generally, the softer the tofu, the lower it is in fat.

A prized attribute of tofu is its versatility. Because it imparts virtually no flavor on its own, its capacity to absorb flavors is heightened. Intermingling flavorfully into any recipe with a variety of textures, tofu is a celebrity in plant-based cooking.

Tofu lends itself to a plethora of possibilities. Silken or soft tofu blends well with other ingredients to become a custard, pudding, or dip. Firm or extra-firm tofu is excellent crumbled into chilies, stews, or scrambles, or cubed and added to stir-fries and soups. With a marinade or herbs and spices, tofu can be baked and served on its own as an entrée.

Traditionally a staple in Indonesia, tempeh is a cultured and fermented soybean cake. Distinguished from tofu by its nutty flavor and chewy texture, tempeh is a delicious, nutrient-dense substitute for meat that's very high in fiber and protein.

Tempeh comes in varieties made with grains, flax, and vegetables and can be used in a variety of ways to add consistency and taste. Crumble tempeh as an alternative to ground meat in a pasta sauce or chili. Slice it, and broil, bake, or stir-fry it with sauce and veggies for a satisfying meal.

When you rinse away all the starch granules from the wheat grain, the protein is left over. This wheat protein, known as gluten, is the basis for a meat analogue called seitan. Prized for its meaty characteristics, seitan is used in hundreds of products that are directly intended to mimic meat.

Plain seitan can be used as a meat alternative when cooked at home with other whole foods. Braised, baked, or cooked in a pressure cooker, seitan works well in stews and sautés.

PLANT PITFALL

Avoid seitan if you have celiac sprue, gluten intolerance, or any wheat allergies or sensitivities.

Commercial items made from seitan include faux shrimp, chicken, shredded pork, and ground round. Inundating the marketplace and vegan restaurants (particularly Asian), seitan exemplifies the intention of a meat analogue.

At home, you can use these seitan-based products as transition foods for the meat-missing members of your family and also as occasional treats. However, be forewarned that most of these foods are processed and contain large amounts of sodium, oil, sugars, and fillers.

Mushrooms

Mushrooms have a hearty, dense mouthfeel similar to meat. Because of their immense nutritional contributions—fiber, folate, copper, potassium, niacin, selenium, riboflavin, and hundreds of phytonutrients—mushrooms make the perfect meat alternative.

Besides their nutrient prowess, mushrooms offer a vast diversity in culinary options. Throw some portobello mushroom caps on the grill for succulent "burgers." Mince mushrooms and use them as you would ground meat in lasagna, stews, casseroles, or sauces. Slice them and add raw to salads, for sushi, or on crudités platters. Scoop out the stems and stuff mushrooms with fillings like nut cheeses, pestos, or vegetable medleys.

MIXED GREENS

Mushrooms are touted for their anticancer and immune-enhancing properties. Used in Eastern medicine in elixirs and teas, mushrooms are high on the list of must-haves in a healthy eating plan.

Un-Cheeses

Now that you know why dairy is best left off your plate and out of your body, it's time to face the repercussions. Cheese has inundated the culinary world with roots deeper than any other food. Besides its addictive properties signaling you to consume more, it's nearly impossible to avoid the presence of cheese in your daily life. Restaurants add cheese to as many dishes as possible. Pizza places work hard to find ways to increase the cheesiness of their products. In television ads, companies go out of their way to provide a tantalizing visual of cheese in their pizzas, burgers, and quesadillas. From these advertisements to the addition of cheese ubiquitously, the allure of cheese is inescapable. You may have grown to love the flavors and textures of cheeses, as most people do.

But after you break your addiction to cheese by abstaining for just a few short weeks, you'll hardly miss it, thanks to myriad plant-based substitutes you can quickly create in your kitchen. With certain flavorings combined with tofu, beans, and other ingredients, you'll never miss cheese again.

If you're not there yet and still need a cheese "crutch," several vegan cheese products are available. These cheese alternatives have really developed over time, and improvements have been made in their melt-ability, flavor, and texture. A couple brands have even been inducted into pizza joints offering plant-based options. In the store, you can now find dairy-free block cheeses, Parmesan flakes, and cheese shreds. Frozen pizzas with vegan cheeses are infiltrating the vast frozen food world as well.

Remember, however, that these products are processed foods. They don't fit the category of whole foods. These faux cheeses still contain oil, sodium, and added flavors. Use them for transition and rare treats only.

A popular favorite in the raw food community is a cheese made of fermented seeds and nuts. Typically, raw sunflower seeds, pumpkin seeds, cashews, pine nuts, macadamia nuts, or almonds are soaked and cultured for a period of a day or two. Preparing these recipes at home enables you to dictate your desired flavors, level of sourness, and consistency.

Blending ingredients like onion powder, garlic powder, miso, and other seasonings with cooked potatoes, chickpeas, or whole-grain flours creates cheesy textures and flavors that satisfy the palate and appease cravings. See Chapter 19 for some examples.

Nutritional Yeast

Although the name might be less than enticing, nutritional yeast is a magnificent staple that will "cheese" up your dishes while providing your daily recommended dose of B vitamins. An excellent source of vitamin B_{12} and protein, nutritional yeast is a primary cultured yeast grown on sugarcane and beet molasses. Unlike other yeasts, it doesn't have leavening power.

The versatility of nutritional yeast is boundless. On its own, it tastes nutty and cheesy and is delicious sprinkled on popcorn. When combined into recipes like hummus, un-cheese spreads, pasta sauce, casseroles, stews, and pizza, nutritional yeast lends a lovely flavor and huge nutrient boost.

You can find nutritional yeast at your local or larger-chain health food stores in tubs by supplements or in the bulk section. Start experimenting, and soon you'll love all the secret beauty in this plant-based essential.

Miso

Salty, pungent, flavor-rich miso is fermented soybean paste usually made in combination with a grain or bean. (It also comes in a soy-free variety made with chickpeas.) Originally from Japan, miso has a rather impressive nutrient report card for a flavoring agent. High in protein, vitamin K, manganese, zinc, and fiber, miso paste boasts the same grade for nutritional value as it does in flavor.

Most famously used to make soup, miso is also delicious as a spread and in dressings, sauces, and sushi. Miso paste provides a zest similar to sharp cheeses and can be blended with other ingredients to create a dairy-free spread. Flavors of miso vary from light and delicate to dark and bold, each offering its own unique flair.

Look for miso in your supermarket's refrigerator section, opting for organic with the soy-based varieties. For some ideas on how to incorporate miso into your diet, try the recipes in Chapters 21 and 22.

Do you see the vastness of the plant-based world? So many delicious ingredients exist that it's impossible to miss your old standards. Maintain your kitchen with a variety of options, and decadent whole-food, plant-based cuisine is always at your fingertips.

The Least You Need to Know

- A well-stocked kitchen enables you to be ready to create, prepare, and consume delicious plant-based foods whenever hunger and creativity strike.
- Essential equipment in the kitchen includes a high-powered blender, a food processor, and a fine set of knives.
- You can effortlessly replace eggs, milk, meats, and cheeses with health-promoting ingredients.
- Certain processed meat alternatives and cheese substitutes make the transition to a plant-based diet easier for some eaters as they move from a plate heavy in animal products to one full of whole-plant foods.

How to Nutrify Any Recipe

In This Chapter

- Honing your nutrification skills
- Manipulating ingredients
- Spicing up your recipes with color, flavor, texture, and nutrients
- Simple substitutions and home-grown tricks

A recipe is a formula of combined ingredients that, ideally, nourishes and satisfies the senses simultaneously. You may have some favorite recipes now but need to improve or adapt them to fit your plant-based diet. No problem.

You need to know how to find beautiful, health-promoting ingredients that are also void of beastly, disease-promoting ones. And, of course, the end product has to be delicious. So you need to identify what needs to change in order to create a nutritious masterpiece. In this chapter, you learn how to inject nutrients into a dish and abolish the antinutrients.

Analyze, Assess, and Amaze Your Friends

You needn't be a chef or have graduated from culinary school to do this. Nor do you have to attain a degree in nutrition to hone your nutrification skills. All you need is an investigative eye, a hungry curiosity, and a smidgen of practice to master this skill.

Instead of narrowing your focus to seek out only whole-food, plant-based recipes, widen your possibilities by learning to nutrify any dish. Train your eyes to discern easily substituted ingredients, and you'll be pleasantly surprised by your options.

Sharpen your skills by practicing, creating, and thinking outside your realm of comfort.

HEALTHY HINT

The best ideas usually emerge by accident. Always keep a pen and paper handy while playing in the kitchen so you can take notes and expand your repertoire every time you learn a new trick.

How many times have you flipped through a cookbook or heard about a new recipe and thought, *Too bad I can't make this because I can't have [fill in the blank]?* It's time to switch to a glass-half-full mentality! A vast plant-based universe with endless choices of ingredients awaits you. With a detective's scrutiny and some creativity, you can master the art and science of plant-based cooking. After all, a great chef is defined not by what he or she can cook, but by what he or she can fix.

Beauty Boosters

What makes a recipe beautiful? A multitude of colors, aromas, flavors, and textures. Nature is bountiful with her infusion of all these characteristics in her plants. Combining them can be magical for both your tongue and your cells.

When analyzing a recipe, identify the power foods—those dense in nutrients, as described in Chapter 4. Greens, beans, other vegetables, fruits, and spices need to take center stage. If not, add them.

Leafy Greens

You can include leafy greens in virtually any dish. Think with your green goggles on whenever preparing any dish to see how you can sneak in more marvelous, leafy green veggies. Here are a few tricks:

- Immediately before your whole-grain pasta is done cooking, add greens to the pot to wilt them. Then drain altogether, and continue with your preparation.

- Stir greens into any type of soup in the form of a vegetable and/or fresh herb. Cilantro perks up Thai- or Latin-flavored soups. Basil makes Italian and Mediterranean soups fresh.

- Boost your salads by adding more than one type of green. In addition to or instead of classic romaine, introduce shredded kale, dandelion greens, and mixed lettuce varieties.

- Include leafy greens in any smoothie or extracted juice you make to enhance nutrients exponentially.

- Spruce up your spreads and dips by processing greens into them for color, flavor, and super nutrition.

- Make ice cream by blending frozen fruit with green cabbage or iceberg lettuce in a high-powered blender.

- Finely chop greens and combine with whole grains such as brown rice or quinoa, some herbs and/or spices, and nutritional yeast for a flavor-rich, nutrient-varied dish.

- Blend greens into stews, stir-fries, casseroles, and sandwiches.

Bountiful Beans

Bring beans back to your dinner plate with gusto. They're as multitalented in the kitchen as they are in your body. With a wide variety of colors, sizes, shapes, textures, and flavors, bump them up in your selection criteria (if you haven't already). Here are a few tips:

- Make fresh beans by cooking them on your stovetop or in a pressure cooker.

- Try bean spreads and dips by processing them with herbs, spices, nutritional yeast, and miso paste (see recipes in Chapter 22).

- Combine beans with grains, stir into soups, and sprinkle on salads.

- Have a bean festival in a pot by making a chili (see recipe in Chapter 21).

HEALTHY HINT

Because beans contain oligosaccharides—sugars that aren't digestible by the human GI tract—they may cause gas in some individuals. To reduce this effect, soak dry beans in water for several hours. Rinse them well before cooking in a fresh batch of water, and add a strip of kombu seaweed to the pot when you start cooking.

Healthful Herbs and Spices

Some herbs and spices have anticancer and antimicrobial properties. They add more than just flavor to your foods!

Used in traditional Chinese and Indian medicine for centuries, turmeric is potent as an anti-inflammatory. It has also been found to contribute anticancer effects, improve liver function, protect the heart, lower cholesterol, and perhaps work against cognitive decline (dementia and Alzheimer's disease). It's even high in iron. Sounds pretty powerful, right?

Turmeric is also easy to consume, with its mild, warm, peppery flavor and bright, staining yellow color. Add turmeric to tofu scrambles to make them yellow, curry dishes, and lentils. Sauté cauliflower, onions, and other vegetables, and stir in turmeric. Whisk it into salad dressings and sauces, and use it to spice up tofu or tempeh salads.

Versatile and pungent, garlic has long been touted for its health advantages. Known as the "stinking rose," garlic acts as an antioxidant, anti-inflammatory, antibacterial, antiviral, antiparasitic, antifungal, and blood thinner. It lowers blood pressure and cholesterol, reduces cancer risk, and improves iron metabolism. When chopped, chewed, or crushed, garlic releases its enzymes and converts the compound alliin into allicin, the active, health-promoting phytonutrient.

Use garlic in spreads, sauces, soups, dressings, sautés, stir-fries, and dips. Roast an unpeeled head at 400°F for about 30 minutes or until the cloves are soft. Peel and spread the garlic on whole-grain breads, tortillas, and crackers. Use this flavor-rich gem to enhance any savory recipe.

Warm and aromatic, zesty and spicy, ginger is a beautiful addition to your ingredient inventory. An effective gastrointestinal reliever, ginger has been used historically to reduce nausea. Ginger also acts as an anti-inflammatory, boosts immunity, and may even prevent cancer by inhibiting the growth of and/or killing cancer cells. Enjoy ginger as a pungent tea, or add it to rice dishes, sauces, dressings, soups, stir-fries, and baked goods.

Cinnamon, a bark that elicits a bite, also has healing capabilities. Cinnamon can improve insulin sensitivity, helping normalize blood sugar levels in diabetics. The oils in cinnamon are antimicrobial and can also inhibit inflammation and blood clotting. Warm up your oatmeal; baked goods; plant milks; pancakes; Indian, Middle Eastern, and African stews; and baked apples with a sprinkle or more of cinnamon.

Speaking of adding warmth, cayenne adds a fiery kick to recipes. Capsaicin is the compound responsible for the heat and health benefits found in cayenne. Another anti-inflammatory, capsaicin also offers relief to those suffering with painful chronic diseases like osteoarthritis, headaches, and diabetic neuropathy. Cayenne clears congestion, boosts immune function, helps dissolve blood clots, decreases cholesterol, and helps you lose weight. Heat up your recipes with a careful dash of cayenne.

HEALTHY HINT

For a warming, spicy treat that also enhances your well-being, make a tea with sliced ginger root and a pinch of cayenne.

Basil is one of the most popular herbs worldwide. Fragrant and familiar, basil is loaded with flavonoids capable of protecting your DNA, and it acts as a potent anti-bacterial agent and anti-inflammatory. Basil is used to make pesto and virtually all Italian dishes. With more than 60 varieties, this versatile herb is a must-have in your kitchen.

Other phytonutrient-dense seasonings include mustard seed, oregano, sage, parsley, rosemary, and onion. Each one offers its own unique personality, lending flavorful undertones to any dish.

Texture Tricks

Besides phytonutrients and seasonings, you can also improve a recipe by influencing textures. In culinary terms, shapes are supposed to stay consistent. If you julienne one vegetable in a dish, you're advised to julienne all the vegetables. This adds to visual and textural appeal.

Create some interest in your dishes by adding chewy to crunchy, soft to firm, dense to light, or thin to thick. Mouthfeel adds a significant layer to food likes and dislikes, so think about varying textures in your dishes. Take tempeh versus tofu, for example. Similar nutritionally and taste-wise, their consistencies are completely different. If you prefer (or just happen to be in the mood for) a smoother, silkier texture, opt to use the tofu. Tempeh is chewier and grainier, satisfying a different mouthfeel.

Experiment with textures as well as flavors, aromas, and colors to get the most out of a recipe. Beautify your plate and your palate with all of nature's gorgeous gifts to stimulate your senses and inspire your culinary competence.

Beast Busters

You should now know what the "beasts" are when it comes to healthful eating. When preparing your own plant-based dishes, find and replace or simply eliminate these ingredients. These include any animal or processed products.

Some recipes are easily nutrified. For example, if you find a chicken stir-fry you're interested in trying, you can simply switch the chicken to tofu, tempeh, or seitan cubes and follow the rest of the recipe.

Of course, not everything is that cut and dried. A steak dinner can be switched for a tempeh steak, but you're better off with a new recipe. In this case, if you can't beat 'em, substitute 'em! Here are some examples:

- Dishes like casseroles and lasagnas are easy to modify. Finely chopped mushrooms, cooked lentils, or crumbled tempeh mimic the mouthfeel of ground meat.

- Swap 1 tablespoon gelatin for 1 tablespoon *agar agar* flakes or ½ teaspoon agar powder (thickens 1 cup liquid).

- Exchange a dairy yogurt with a soy- or rice-based version. Be wary of sugar-filled products. Instead, buy the plain flavor, and add fresh fruit and date paste for a whole-food version. Plain plant-based yogurt works well as a moisture-adding ingredient in baking. It can also add a creamy texture when cooking sauces, curries, or soups.

- Make buttermilk by adding 2 teaspoons lemon juice or white vinegar to 1 cup soy milk.

- Vegetable broth can easily replace chicken, meat, or fish broth. For a meatier flavor, add tamari or miso paste to water or vegetable broth to taste.

- For frozen desserts, choose whole-fruit sorbet or popsicles, or blend frozen fruit in a high-powered blender.

DEFINITION

Agar agar is a gelatinous substance derived from seaweed that works as a thickening agent and can replace gelatin as a plant-based substitute.

Hundreds of products free of animal ingredients are currently on the market, such as sour cream, butter, mayonnaise, whipped cream, ice cream, creamer, mock meats, cheese, and cream cheese. Although these goods are a step up in terms of harmfulness, they're still processed foods. Oils, sugars, sodium, added flavors, and colors are used to mimic the original versions. Instead of allowing these items to populate your daily diet, position them at the very tiptop of the Plant-Based Food Guide Pyramid, and use them sparingly.

If you have a serious medical condition like diabetes, heart disease, or cancer, stay away from the processed foods entirely to allow your body to gain maximum benefit from whole-food, plant-based nutrition. Moderation is inadequate when your body needs to heal and recover. You need to keep your diet at the highest level of purity and nourish yourself properly.

You can look at vegan recipes for a ton of ideas, too. To convert a vegan recipe into a whole-food recipe, use these simple substitutions:

- Replace oil in cooking with equal amounts of water, vegetable broth, vinegar, wine, or beer. In baking, replace 1 cup oil with 1 cup applesauce or other fruit purée (such as pumpkin, banana, squash, or prunes).

- Swap salt for kelp powder in equal amounts. (You may need more kelp powder if you're still used to eating high amounts of salt.) You can also use salt-free seasonings found in the store or online.

- For any sweetening, use dates or date paste (see the next section for how to make your own) or 100 percent pure maple syrup.

DIY Ingredients

You can easily whip up several ingredients at home, providing you with 100 percent whole-food options. These quickies are a superior investment and save you from apprehension and label-reading time—and also provide better taste.

Date Paste

Date paste is the ultimate sweetener. This easy DIY whole food can replace sugars in baking and add sweetness to dressings, smoothies, and sauces.

Dates
Water or unsweetened almond milk

1. Soak dates in water or unsweetened almond milk for several hours to soften. Add only enough liquid to cover dates so your end paste isn't too thin.

2. When dates appear flaky and swollen, pour off a little liquid. In a blender or food processor, blend remaining liquid with dates for 1 or 2 minutes or until smooth, stopping to scrape down the sides as needed.

HEALTHY HINT

If you're in a rush or decide to make a recipe with date paste before you've had time to soak the dates, use hot water to expedite the process.

Parmesan Shake

Who needs dairy when you can make this plant-perfect Parmesan shake in less than a minute?

1 cup raw almonds	4 TB. raw sesame seeds
1 cup nutritional yeast flakes	2 tsp. kelp powder

1. Add almonds, nutritional yeast flakes, sesame seeds, and kelp powder to a food processor, and process for 45 to 60 seconds or until mixture turns into a powder.

2. Use on everything from pasta dishes and lasagnas, to salads, soups, spreads, dips, casseroles, and anywhere else you'd use the dairy version.

MIXED GREENS

This shake is high in calcium, magnesium, vitamin E, all the B vitamins, protein, and healthy fats. Best of all, you avoid the saturated fat, cholesterol, sodium, and other no-no's in the original version.

Plant-Based Sour Cream

Sour cream can be nutrified and taste even better than store-bought when you make it at home with whole-plant foods.

14 oz. silken tofu	2 TB. nutritional yeast flakes
¼ cup unsweetened soy milk	1½ tsp. kelp powder
4 TB. freshly squeezed lemon juice	1 TB. chopped fresh parsley or 1 tsp. dried parsley flakes (optional)

1. In a food processor, combine tofu, soy milk, lemon juice, nutritional yeast flakes, kelp powder, and parsley for 2 minutes or until smooth.

2. Keep tightly covered in the refrigerator for 3 or 4 days.

You can also save some bucks by making your own flours. Simply grind away whole grains like oats and buckwheat in a high-powered blender until the mixture is fine and powdery.

Or you can make nut flour by processing raw nuts alone or in combination. (And if you find you've overprocessed the nuts, enjoy your homemade nut butter!) Nut flours are great for dessert bases like pie crusts, cookies, and bars. They provide dense nutrition along with rich flavor. Process them with dried fruit for a homemade nutrition bar.

A new perspective breeds creativity. Challenge and excite yourself to explore, mix, match, blend, and combine. Avoiding and substituting the beasts has never been so easy. Take some time investigating products and ingredients. Focus on Mother Nature's boundless beauties to add color, texture, and flavor in ways that may be new to you. You never know what you may discover!

The Least You Need to Know

- Be on the lookout for ways to sneak more power foods like leafy green veggies, beans, herbs, and spices into your meals.
- Many recipes can be easily converted to whole-food, plant-based versions by avoiding animal and processed foods as main ingredients.

- Nutrify your favorite recipes by substituting whole-plant food ingredients for the originals. Homemade imitation products like sour cream, Parmesan cheese, and date paste taste superior to the original, processed versions.
- One of the easiest ways to create a new work of genius is to take a vegan recipe and substitute the oil and/or sweeteners with a whole-food version.
- Have fun playing with plant-based ingredients. You have nothing to lose and only delicious cuisine and ingenious culinary tricks to gain!

Morning, Noon, and Light Fare

In This Chapter

- Delicious breakfast starters
- Delightful early day options
- Bright and colorful lunches

Some people take breakfast very seriously, while others blow it off due to a rushed schedule or lack of hunger. Regardless of your position, your first meal should be gentle and nutrient-rich because this is when you're breaking your overnight fast. Your cells are hungry and receptive to nourishment. Whether you're rushed or have time for a more leisurely morning meal, the recipes in this chapter provide you with a huge nutritional boost.

All these breakfast and lunch options travel well. Find a huge smoothie mug for a daily on-the-go green smoothie in the morning. Make the soup or dressings the night before to save time in the morning. No matter how rushed the early part of your day is, be sure to take time to smell the spinach!

It's Easy Being Green Smoothie

Fruity and sweet, frosty and creamy, this smoothie is so delectable.

Yield:	Prep time:	Serving size:	
6 cups	10 minutes	1 smoothie	
Each serving has:			
460 calories	13g total fat	0.5g saturated fat	0g trans fat
0mg cholesterol	460mg sodium	82g total carbohydrates	20g dietary fiber
46g sugars	11g protein	536mg calcium	5mg iron

4 cups packed green leafy vegetables (spinach, dandelion greens, collard greens, kale, and/or other favorite greens)

2 TB. hempseeds and/or flaxseeds

1 cup frozen blueberries

¼ cup frozen cherries

¼ cup frozen raspberries

¼ cup frozen pineapple pieces

¼ cup frozen mango chunks

1 medium frozen peeled banana, broken into pieces

2 cups unsweetened almond milk

1. In a high-powered blender, combine greens, hempseeds, blueberries, cherries, raspberries, pineapple, mango, banana, and almond milk.

2. Blend on high speed for 60 seconds or until smooth. Enjoy icy cold.

Variation: You can substitute 2 cups *coconut water*, cooled green tea, or other plant milk for the almond milk.

DEFINITION

Coconut water, the clear liquid found inside a young coconut, is extremely high in electrolytes and makes an excellent natural sports drink.

Mint Chocolate Nib Smoothie

Minty, sweet, and decadent, this breakfast smoothie will refresh and energize you.

Yield:	Prep time:	Serving size:	
5 cups	5 minutes	2½ cups	
Each serving has:			
450 calories	13g total fat	4g saturated fat	0g trans fat
0mg cholesterol	230mg sodium	80g total carbohydrates	25g dietary fiber
35g sugars	12g protein	356mg calcium	9mg iron

3 cups packed green leafy vegetables (spinach, dandelion greens, collard greens, kale, and/or other favorite greens)

1 cup fresh mint leaves, chopped

2 TB. hempseeds and/or flaxseeds

6 medium pitted dates

½ cup raw cacao nibs

1 cup frozen blueberries

2 medium frozen peeled bananas, broken into pieces

1 cup ice

2 cups unsweetened chocolate almond milk

1. In a high-powered blender, combine greens, mint, hempseeds, dates, cacao nibs, blueberries, bananas, ice, and almond milk.

2. Blend on high speed for 60 seconds or until smooth. Enjoy icy cold.

Variation: If this smoothie isn't sweet enough for you, add more dates to suit your taste.

HEALTHY HINT

Challenge yourself to pack the blender with more and more greens as your taste buds evolve through the plant-based world.

Chocolate Almond Butter in a Cup

Rich and dreamy, this candy-in-a-glass green smoothie will put a smile on your face.

Yield:	Prep time:	Serving size:	
4 cups	5 minutes	2 cups	
Each serving has:			
590 calories	30g total fat	4.5g saturated fat	0g trans fat
0mg cholesterol	230mg sodium	74g total carbohydrates	23g dietary fiber
30g sugars	19g protein	374mg calcium	5mg iron

4 cups fresh spinach, tightly packed

¼ cup raw almond butter

2 TB. hempseeds and/or flaxseeds

6 pitted dates

½ cup raw cacao nibs

2 medium frozen peeled bananas, broken into pieces

1 cup ice

2 cups unsweetened chocolate almond milk

1. In a high-powered blender, place spinach, almond butter, hempseeds, dates, cacao nibs, bananas, ice, and almond milk.

2. Blend on high speed for 60 seconds or until smooth. Enjoy icy cold.

Variation: Feel free to use a different raw nut butter in place of the almond butter. Try ¼ cup unsweetened peanut butter or cashew butter instead.

HEALTHY HINT

You can make your own nut butter by processing raw nuts and/or seeds in your food processor until pasty.

Blueberry Banana Pancakes

Hearty and syrupy, these fruity pancakes make a great weekend morning treat.

Yield:	Prep time:	Cook time:	Serving size:
4 large pancakes	10 minutes	10 minutes	2 large pancakes
Each serving has:			
190 calories	2g total fat	0g saturated fat	0g trans fat
0mg cholesterol	40mg sodium	40g total carbohydrates	6g dietary fiber
13g sugars	7g protein	611mg calcium	2mg iron

1 medium banana	2 tsp. baking powder
¼ cup plant milk (almond, soy, oat)	1 TB. pure maple syrup
1 cup whole-grain flour (oat, whole-wheat, etc.)	1 cup fresh or thawed frozen blueberries

1. In a large bowl, mash banana with a fork. Add plant milk and mix until lump-free.

2. Add whole-grain flour and baking powder to banana mixture, and mix with a fork just until dry ingredients are moistened. Stir in maple syrup and blueberries until incorporated.

3. Heat a medium skillet over medium-high heat until hot. Pour ½ cup batter into the skillet. Reduce heat to medium, and cover. Cook for 2 to 4 minutes or until pancake starts to brown at the edge. Using a spatula, turn pancake and cook other side for 1 or 2 minutes or until golden brown. Repeat with remaining batter.

4. Drizzle with additional maple syrup, if desired, to serve.

MIXED GREENS

Whole-grain flour mixes are available commercially. You can probably even find gluten-free options easily. Experiment with different varieties to see which you prefer.

Veggie Tofu Scramble

This scramble offers skillet-sizzled classic tastes. Buttery and silky, the garlicky, onion bite will induce long-term cravings.

Yield:	Prep time:	Cook time:	Serving size:
4 cups	10 minutes	12 to 16 minutes	1 cup
Each serving has:			
140 calories	4.5g total fat	0g saturated fat	0g trans fat
0mg cholesterol	470mg sodium	10g total carbohydrates	3g dietary fiber
2g sugars	14g protein	174mg calcium	3mg iron

1 small yellow onion, chopped

5 medium baby bella mushrooms, sliced

¼ cup vegetable broth

1 (12-oz.) pkg. firm or extra-firm tofu, drained and crumbled

1 TB. tamari

1 TB. dried parsley flakes

1 TB. nutritional yeast flakes

½ tsp. garlic powder

½ tsp. onion powder

½ tsp. turmeric

½ tsp. freshly ground black pepper

1 cup chopped fresh spinach

½ cup salsa

1. In a medium saucepan over medium heat, sauté onions and mushrooms in vegetable broth for 5 minutes or until onions are translucent.

2. Stir in tofu, tamari, dried parsley flakes, nutritional yeast flakes, garlic powder, onion powder, turmeric, and black pepper, and simmer for 10 to 12 minutes or until moisture has evaporated. Add spinach and salsa, and scramble for 2 to 4 more minutes or until brown at the edges.

3. Serve hot with warmed corn tortillas or a side of brown rice or quinoa, if desired.

MIXED GREENS

Dried mushrooms have an intense, rich, umami flavor that can be used in many different ways. Grind them into a powder, and sprinkle it into soups, casseroles, or stews as a seasoning. Or reconstitute them for use as you would fresh mushrooms.

Breakfast Rice Pudding

Knowing this cozy and enticing pudding is on the menu, you'll love waking up on a cold day. The cinnamon undertones are warming, while the crunch of the smooth almonds mixed with the chewiness of the raisins makes this dish hearty.

Yield:	Prep time:	Cook time:	Serving size:
6 cups	5 minutes	20 minutes	1½ cups
Each serving has:			
420 calories	11g total fat	1g saturated fat	0g trans fat
0mg cholesterol	70mg sodium	72g total carbohydrates	6g dietary fiber
36g sugars	12g protein	304mg calcium	3mg iron

2 cups cooked brown rice	1 TB. alcohol-free vanilla extract
1 cup raisins	1 TB. ground cinnamon
½ cup slivered raw almonds	3 cups unsweetened soy milk
¼ cup pure maple syrup	

1. In a medium saucepan over medium heat, combine brown rice, raisins, raw almonds, maple syrup, vanilla extract, ground cinnamon, and soy milk.

2. Bring to a boil, and reduce heat to low. Simmer over low heat, stirring occasionally, for 20 minutes or until pudding thickens.

3. Serve hot, or refrigerate to serve chilled.

HEALTHY HINT

This pudding is the perfect dish to use up your leftover rice. Or in a pinch, microwave single-ingredient ready-cooked brown rice packets to use instead.

Japanese Noritos

Crispy nori sheets make for a delightfully light wrapper, surrounding the crunchy and savory filling. Blending these textures will remind you of sushi but with a heartier feel.

Yield:	Prep time:	Serving size:	
2 noritos	10 minutes	2 noritos	
Each serving has:			
140 calories	2g total fat	0g saturated fat	0g trans fat
0mg cholesterol	460mg sodium	20g total carbohydrates	4g dietary fiber
2g sugars	6g protein	62mg calcium	1mg iron

2 sheets nori	1½ TB. shredded carrots
1 tsp. low-sodium miso paste	1 tsp. tamari
¼ cup cooked brown rice	1 tsp. sesame seeds or gomashio
½ small *Persian cucumber,* julienned	

1. Place nori sheets on a flat surface. Gently and evenly place miso paste on ½ of each nori sheet.

2. Add brown rice, Persian cucumber, and shredded carrots on top of miso paste. Drizzle with tamari, and lightly sprinkle sesame seeds over top.

3. Tightly roll nori like a burrito from ingredient-filled side.

Variation: For **Mexican Noritos,** substitute filling with 3 tablespoons Sweet Pea Guacamole (recipe in Chapter 22), ¼ cup julienned jicama, ½ tablespoon chopped fresh cilantro, and 2 tablespoons salsa.

DEFINITION

The word ***norito*** is a combination of *nori* and *burrito,* because these rolls, filled with crunchy and savory filling and wrapped in crispy nori sheets, ultimately end up looking, and being eaten, like burritos. **Persian cucumbers** are mini seedless cucumbers that are crisp, refreshing, and available throughout the year.

Holy Kale with Herbed Tahini Dressing

You won't be able to stop eating oh-so-good-for-you kale after you try this fresh, sweet, and herbed delightful dressing. Rich and creamy, zesty and nutty, the garlic and cilantro tones will make you an instant fan.

Yield:	Prep time:	Serving size:	
12 cups	20 minutes	2 cups	
Each serving has:			
270 calories	8g total fat	<1g saturated fat	0g trans fat
0mg cholesterol	252mg sodium	43g total carbohydrates	5g dietary fiber
8g sugars	13g protein	353mg calcium	5mg iron

10 cups curly kale, rinsed, drained, and shredded	¼ cup freshly squeezed lime juice
1 cup carrots, shredded	1 TB. lime zest
1 cup red cabbage, shredded	6 pitted dates
1 (15-oz.) can cannellini beans, rinsed and drained	3 TB. tahini
1 cup water	3 TB. hempseeds
1½ cups fresh cilantro, de-stemmed	2 TB. tamari
1 cup fresh Italian parsley, de-stemmed	1 large clove garlic, peeled and crushed
	½ tsp. cayenne

1. In a large salad bowl, combine kale, carrots, and red cabbage.

2. In a blender, combine cannellini beans, water, cilantro, Italian parsley, lime juice, lime zest, dates, tahini, hempseeds, tamari, garlic, and cayenne. Blend on high speed for 1 minute or until creamy and smooth.

3. Pour dressing over salad, toss to evenly distribute, and serve immediately.

Variation: You can substitute 1½ cups other fresh herbs like dill or basil for the cilantro. Either way, the herbed tahini dressing is also delicious on any vegetable salad or over a baked potato.

PLANT PITFALL

Only zest citrus fruits that are organically grown or washed carefully with soap and water first. Citrus rind has a tendency to hold onto a lot of pesticide and other chemical residues on its surface.

Sushi Salad with Creamy Miso Dressing

Free-style sushi all in a big bowl, this salad is refreshingly crisp and fulfilling, with gingery, pungent, and peppery flavors from the East.

Yield:	Prep time:	Serving size:	
8 cups	30 minutes	1⅓ cups	
Each serving has:			
180 calories	9g total fat	1g saturated fat	0g trans fat
0mg cholesterol	70mg sodium	21g total carbohydrates	6g dietary fiber
4g sugars	6g protein	43mg calcium	1mg iron

4 sheets *nori*	½ cup water
1 cup cooked brown rice	2 TB. raw tahini
2 cups chopped romaine lettuce	3 pitted dates
1 cup shredded red cabbage	1 TB. low-sodium miso paste
1 cup shredded carrots	3 TB. freshly squeezed lemon juice
1 cup julienned cucumbers	1 TB. unsweetened rice vinegar
1 cup frozen shelled edamame, thawed	1 tsp. minced fresh ginger
	1 medium clove garlic, minced
1 medium avocado, peeled, pitted, and sliced	⅓ tsp. red chili flakes
	¼ tsp. Chinese five-spice powder (optional)
1 TB. pickled ginger (optional)	

1. On a cutting board, use a pair of scissors to shred nori sheets into pieces. Line up nori sheets around the perimeter of a large bowl to create a border. Spoon brown rice into the center. Pile romaine lettuce, red cabbage, carrots, cucumbers, and edamame on top of rice.

2. Gently place avocado on the top, and add pickled ginger (if using) in the center.

3. In a high-powered blender or food processor, combine water, tahini, dates, miso paste, lemon juice, rice vinegar, ginger, garlic, chili flakes, and Chinese five-spice powder (if using). Blend or process for 1 minute or until dressing is smooth and creamy.

4. Toss dressing and salad, and serve.

DEFINITION

Nori, the Japanese name for seaweed, is dried, typically toasted, made into flat sheets, and used as a sushi wrapper.

Zel's Zesty Rainbow Salad

A lightly spiced, herb-based dressing, boosted with the nutritional benefits of nuts, tempers the distinct flavor of cilantro in this salad for the perfect balance of tang and tastiness.

Yield:	Prep time:	Serving size:	
8 cups	30 to 45 minutes	1⅓ cups	
Each serving has:			
140 calories	5g total fat	1g saturated fat	0g trans fat
0mg cholesterol	210mg sodium	19g total carbohydrates	5g dietary fiber
5g sugars	7g protein	99mg calcium	2mg iron

1 large head broccoli, cut into bite-size pieces

1 medium bunch watercress, coarsely chopped

8 medium leaves romaine lettuce, coarsely shredded

2 or 3 medium carrots, coarsely shredded

2 cups frozen peas, thawed

1½ cups shredded red cabbage

4 to 6 medium radishes, sliced

1 small whole green onion

2 cups coarsely chopped fresh cilantro, lightly packed

1 cup water

½ cup cashews or macadamia nuts

¼ cup white wine vinegar

3 TB. fresh lemon juice

2 medium cloves garlic, minced

2 tsp. red miso

¾ tsp. ground cumin

½ tsp. ground coriander

½ tsp. lemon pepper

½ tsp. guar gum or xanthan gum

Pinch cayenne

1. Fill a 3-quart saucepan ⅔ full with water, and bring to a boil over high heat. In small batches, blanch broccoli for 1 minute. Using a slotted spoon, remove broccoli to a dish or bowl to cool. Repeat with remaining broccoli pieces, and set aside.

2. In a large salad bowl, toss watercress and lettuce. Pile cooled broccoli into the center, heaping it high.

3. Surround broccoli with a circle of shredded carrots, followed by a circle of peas, filling the entire surface and covering greens.

4. Arrange red cabbage in 4 piles over peas, and place sliced radishes in spaces between cabbage. Artfully place green onion near center of salad.

5. In a blender, combine cilantro, 1 cup water, cashews, white wine vinegar, lemon juice, garlic, red miso, cumin, coriander, lemon pepper, guar gum, and cayenne. Blend on high speed for 60 seconds or until fully puréed and dressing is smooth and creamy.

6. Pour dressing into a narrow-neck bottle for easy serving. Shake well before serving with salad. (Refrigerated, dressing will keep for 1 week.)

MIXED GREENS

Salads ought to be colorful and so visually appealing they're irresistible, luring diners to the table. The salad's health benefits are a bonus.

Cream of Carrot Soup

This bright-orange, delicately aromatic soup imparts a sweetness and tang that goes down smoothly.

Yield:	Prep time:	Cook time:	Serving size:
8 cups	5 minutes	15 to 20 minutes	2 cups
Each serving has:			
100 calories	1.5g total fat	0g saturated fat	0g trans fat
0mg cholesterol	640mg sodium	18g total carbohydrates	5g dietary fiber
9g sugars	4g protein	145mg calcium	1mg iron

8 large carrots, chopped

4 cups vegetable broth

1 cup unsweetened soy milk

1 TB. chopped fresh dill or 1 tsp. dried dillweed

½ tsp. freshly ground black pepper

1½ TB. tamari

1. In a large soup pot over medium heat, simmer carrots in vegetable broth for 15 to 20 minutes or until carrots become tender.

2. Add soy milk, dill, black pepper, and tamari. Using an immersion bender, blend on high speed until slightly chunky or smooth, depending on your preference.

3. Serve hot.

HEALTHY HINT

If you don't have an immersion blender, carefully pour ingredients into a regular blender to purée. Return soup to the pot after it's blended.

Cold Melon Soup

This all-raw ingredient soup is refreshing during hot summer months when juicy, sweet, overly ripe melons offer the best flavor.

Yield:	Prep time:	Serving size:	
6 cups	5 to 7 minutes	1 cup	
Each serving has:			
70 calories	0g total fat	0g saturated fat	0g trans fat
0mg cholesterol	25mg sodium	17g total carbohydrates	2g dietary fiber
15g sugars	2g protein	19mg calcium	0mg iron

2 lb. cantaloupe or other melon, peeled and cut into cubes

2 cups water

Juice of 2 oranges

Juice of 2 limes

1 TB. minced fresh ginger

1. In a high-powered blender, combine cantaloupe, water, orange juice, lime juice, and ginger.

2. Blend for 2 or 3 minutes or until completely smooth. Transfer to a glass bowl, and serve immediately, or cover and chill in the refrigerator for 1 hour or more.

Variation: To create other fruit soups, replace the cantaloupe with an equal amount of nectarines, peaches, or a combination of other fresh fruits or berries. For a lighter soup, add ½ cup soy yogurt or nondairy milk of choice.

HEALTHY HINT

With a mere single cup of cantaloupe, you can get your entire day's worth of both vitamin C and vitamin A!

Dinner Delights

In This Chapter

- International noodle dishes
- Classic legume and grain combos
- Hearty herbaceous helpings

A proper dinner involves sitting relaxingly at the table after a long, productive day, slowly savoring a delicious, nutritious meal. Yet this isn't always the case.

Some of the recipes in this chapter are quick and simple, while others yield large batches so you can refrigerate or even freeze the leftovers for future dinners when you may be too tired or pressed for time to cook. Supplementing with salads and soups and/or mixing and matching for a sample-style meal works great to enhance variety and satiate your hunger.

The recipes in this chapter, from all around the world, are dinner staples in my house. I sometimes even eat them for breakfast (but shhh, don't tell anyone!).

Japanoodles

Miso adds a savory, salty component that, together with garlic and sesame, provides the perfect amount of flavor to coat the silky rice noodles.

Yield:	Prep time:	Cook time:	Serving size:
4 cups	5 minutes	5 minutes	1 cup
Each serving has:			
290 calories	1g total fat	0g saturated fat	0g trans fat
0mg cholesterol	710mg sodium	56g total carbohydrates	2g dietary fiber
0g sugars	6g protein	80mg calcium	1mg iron

4 qt. water

1 (8-oz.) pkg. dry rice noodles

½ cup low-sodium miso paste

2 or 3 medium cloves garlic, crushed

2 tsp. *gomashio* or sesame seeds

4 cups chopped mixed leafy green vegetables (chard, dandelion greens, collard greens, spinach, and/or kale)

1. In a medium saucepan over medium-high heat, bring water to a boil. Add rice noodles and boil for 4 or 5 minutes.

2. Meanwhile, in a large bowl, mix together miso paste, garlic, and gomashio.

3. About 30 seconds before noodles are done, add greens to the pan and allow to wilt. Drain noodles and greens in a colander.

4. Add noodles and greens to miso paste mixture, and stir to combine. Serve warm.

DEFINITION

Gomashio is a Japanese condiment made of a blend of toasted sesame seeds, salt, and sometimes sea vegetables.

Herbed Balsamic Pasta

Garden-fresh herbs complemented by balsamic zest inspire the feel of a stroll through Tuscany—an altogether satisfying Italian experience.

Yield:	Prep time:	Serving size:	
6 cups	20 minutes	1½ cups	
Each serving has:			
280 calories	1.5g total fat	0g saturated fat	0g trans fat
0mg cholesterol	40mg sodium	58g total carbohydrates	5g dietary fiber
5g sugars	8g protein	57mg calcium	2mg iron

4 qt. water	1 TB. minced fresh or 1 tsp. dried rosemary
1 (12-oz.) pkg. whole-grain pasta	Pinch sea salt (optional)
1½ cups chopped fresh basil	¾ tsp. freshly ground black pepper
1 TB. minced fresh or 1 tsp. dried oregano	½ cup balsamic vinegar
	2 cups chopped fresh spinach

1. In a medium pot over medium-high heat, bring water to a boil. Add pasta and cook according to the package directions.

2. Meanwhile, in a large bowl, combine basil, oregano, rosemary, sea salt (if using), black pepper, and balsamic vinegar.

3. About 1 minute before pasta is done cooking (test it to be sure it's soft), add spinach to the pot with pasta.

4. After 1 minute maximum, drain pasta and spinach in a colander. Add to balsamic vinegar mixture and toss well, coating pasta adequately. Serve warm.

PLANT PITFALL

If you're salt-sensitive or have been diagnosed with high blood pressure or kidney disease, omit the salt called for in recipes.

Easy Beans and Quinoa

This warm and hearty one-pot wonder has a very Southwestern flare.

Yield:	Prep time:	Cook time:	Serving size:
4 cups	10 minutes	30 minutes	1 cup

Each serving has:			
170 calories	2g total fat	0g saturated fat	0g trans fat
0mg cholesterol	180mg sodium	30g total carbohydrates	6g dietary fiber
2g sugars	8g protein	64mg calcium	3mg iron

1 small yellow onion, chopped	1 cup water
2 medium cloves garlic, minced or crushed	½ tsp. ground cumin
¼ cup vegetable broth	¼ tsp. sea salt (optional)
½ cup dry quinoa	¼ tsp. freshly ground black pepper
1 (15-oz.) can no-salt-added pinto or black beans, rinsed and drained	½ cup frozen corn kernels, thawed
	¼ cup chopped fresh cilantro

1. In a medium pot over medium heat, sauté onion and garlic in vegetable broth for 5 minutes or until onions are translucent.

2. Add quinoa, pinto beans, water, cumin, sea salt (if using), and black pepper. Bring to a boil, lower heat to low, and simmer for 20 minutes, stirring frequently, or until all liquid is absorbed.

3. Stir in corn and cilantro until heated through. Remove from heat and serve.

MIXED GREENS

Cilantro is actually the stems and leaves of the coriander plant. Popular in the Southwestern and Western regions of the United States, cilantro has a pungent odor many people don't appreciate. Italian parsley can be used instead of cilantro if you're not a fan.

Baked Lentils and Rice Casserole

Rustic and hearty, this simple baked dish will be a regular staple in your home.

Yield:	Prep time:	Cook time:	Serving size:
10 cups	5 minutes	90 minutes	1¾ cups

Each serving has:			
250 calories	1g total fat	0g saturated fat	0g trans fat
0mg cholesterol	190mg sodium	48g total carbohydrates	14g dietary fiber
3g sugars	13g protein	66mg calcium	4mg iron

1 medium yellow onion, chopped	1 TB. chopped fresh or 1 tsp. dried rosemary
1 cup uncooked wild and/or brown rice	1 TB. chopped fresh or 1 tsp. dried basil
1 cup dried lentils (red, green, and/or caviar)	1 tsp. chopped fresh or 1 tsp. dried oregano
1 (14-oz.) can crushed tomatoes, with juice	4 cups vegetable broth

1. Preheat the oven to 350°F.

2. In a large, deep baking dish, combine onion, rice, lentils, tomatoes, rosemary, basil, oregano, and vegetable broth, and stir gently.

3. Bake, covered, for 90 minutes, stirring every 30 minutes to prevent sticking, until bubbling and browned. Serve warm.

MIXED GREENS

Lentils are one of the most nutrient-dense foods around. With loads of fiber, protein, iron, and folate, these nutritional superstars will rock your world!

Versatile Bean Sauté

Warm with a hearty Middle Eastern spicy kick, this recipe is quick and yet so satisfying.

Yield:	Prep time:	Cook time:	Serving size:
2 cups	10 minutes	10 minutes	1 cup

Each serving has:			
250 calories	2g total fat	0g saturated fat	0g trans fat
0mg cholesterol	640mg sodium	48g total carbohydrates	10g dietary fiber
3g sugars	10g protein	95mg calcium	4mg iron

1 small red onion, chopped	1 medium tomato, chopped
2 TB. vegetable broth	1 tsp. ground cumin
1 (15-oz.) can chickpeas, rinsed and drained	1 tsp. turmeric
	Freshly ground black pepper

1. In a medium saucepan over medium heat, sauté red onion in vegetable broth for 5 minutes or until onion is translucent.

2. Add chickpeas, tomato, cumin, turmeric, and black pepper, and stir with a wooden spoon for 5 minutes or until heated through. Serve immediately.

Variation: Consider vegifying this recipe by adding any chopped raw veggies you have in your fridge, such as mushrooms, bell peppers, spinach, broccoli, cauliflower, summer squash, or eggplant.

HEALTHY HINT

This dish is a great staple and can be used in a variety of ways. Serve it over steamed brown rice or quinoa for a more substantial meal. Top a salad with it for heartiness. Or plate it onto a baked potato.

Steamed Veggie Sampler

Steaming vegetables until they're just crisp-tender is one of the healthiest ways to prepare them because it preserves more of the nutrients than boiling or oven-roasting. Tossed with fresh herbs and a little vegetable broth, and given a squeeze of fresh lemon juice at the end, perks up their naturally sweet and unique flavors.

Yield:	Prep time:	Cook time:	Serving size:
6 cups	10 to 15 minutes	8 to 15 minutes	1 cup

Each serving has:			
45 calories	0g total fat	0g saturated fat	0g trans fat
0mg cholesterol	40mg sodium	9g total carbohydrates	2g dietary fiber
3g sugars	3g protein	47mg calcium	1mg iron

4 large cloves garlic, peeled	¼ cup low-sodium vegetable broth
1½ cups small cauliflower florets	¼ cup chopped fresh parsley
1½ cups small broccoli florets	1 TB. chopped fresh dill or thyme, or to taste
1 cup (¼-in.-thick) diagonally cut carrots or diagonally halved baby carrots	Sea salt
1 cup sugar snap peas, ends trimmed	Freshly ground black pepper
1½ cups (2-in.-long) diagonally cut asparagus, ends trimmed	1 lemon, cut into wedges

1. In a large pot with a collapsible steamer basket or a steamer rack insert, add garlic and set over medium-high heat. Add enough water so it just touches the bottom of the collapsible steamer, or add 1 or 2 inches water if using a rack insert (garlic should not come into direct contact with the water). Cover and bring to a boil.

2. Depending on the steamer setup, steam vegetables separately in batches or all together. Cauliflower and broccoli florets take 5 to 7 minutes, carrots and sugar snap peas take 3 to 5 minutes, and asparagus takes 2 or 3 minutes to steam. If steaming all together, add them in order, starting with cauliflower and broccoli florets, after 2 minutes add carrots and sugar snap peas, and when they're crisp-tender, add asparagus and steam for 2 minutes.

3. Transfer steamed vegetables to a large bowl. Remove garlic cloves from water with a slotted spoon, slice or chop, and add to steamed vegetables, if desired.

4. Add vegetable broth, parsley, dill, sea salt, and black pepper, and toss well to combine. Squeeze fresh lemon juice over individual servings, and serve hot.

Variation: Feel free to substitute other vegetables in this recipe such as potatoes, turnips, artichokes, Brussels sprouts, green beans, corn, greens, mushrooms, or zucchini that have been cut into bite-size pieces and steamed until crisp-tender. Omit fresh herbs and vegetable broth, if desired, and instead season with sea salt and black pepper to serve with your favorite vinaigrette or creamy salad dressing.

HEALTHY HINT

When steaming, be sure to use a pot that's large enough to hold items and allows the steam to fully circulate around them. Be sure the water is boiling and producing steam before adding the vegetables, and keep the pot tightly covered to prevent the steam from escaping. When removing the lid, lean back to avoid being burned by the steam, and use pot holders to remove the steamer basket or insert. Finally, you can use the liquid that remains in the pot to flavor soups, stews, and sauces.

Fiesta Fantastica

The earthy spices enrich the warm, hearty lentils and are contrasted by fresh crisp greens and all the blended flavors of the accoutrements.

Yield:	Prep time:	Cook time:	Serving size:
4 tostadas	10 minutes	55 minutes	1 tostada
Each serving has:			
340 calories	10g total fat	1.5g saturated fat	0g trans fat
0mg cholesterol	740mg sodium	52g total carbohydrates	14g dietary fiber
5g sugars	16g protein	125mg calcium	4mg iron

1 medium yellow onion, chopped

2 medium cloves garlic, crushed

3 cups vegetable broth

1 cup green lentils, dried and rinsed

1 tsp. ground cumin

1 tsp. turmeric

1 tsp. freshly ground black pepper

1 tsp. chili powder

4 large or 8 small whole-grain tortillas

4 cups chopped mixed greens

1 cup Sweet Pea Guacamole (recipe in Chapter 22)

1 cup Plant-Based Sour Cream (recipe in Chapter 19)

1 cup oil-free, low-sodium salsa

1. In a medium saucepan over medium heat, sauté onions and garlic in ¼ cup vegetable broth for 5 minutes or until onions are translucent.

2. Add lentils, cumin, turmeric, black pepper, chili powder, and remaining 2¾ cups vegetable broth. Simmer for 40 to 50 minutes or until all liquid is absorbed.

3. Warm tortillas on the stovetop, in the microwave, or in a toaster oven until heated through. Spoon lentils onto tortillas, and layer mixed greens, Sweet Pea Guacamole, Plant-Based Sour Cream, and salsa on top. Serve immediately.

Variations: For more of a taco or burrito, use less stuffing and roll it up. To make a **Fiesta Fantastica Salad Extraordinaire,** add more raw veggie strips like cucumbers, bell peppers, tomatoes, and jicama.

HEALTHY HINT

When shopping for salsa, why not try one of the delicious commercially prepared salsas available? You can find sweet, fruit-based salsas (like peach or mango), ones with added beans, and freshly made salsas stocked in the produce section of many supermarkets.

Wacky Wild Rice

With its Mediterranean flavors and mixture of textures, this grainy, slightly acidic rice dish hits the spot.

Yield:	Prep time:	Cook time:	Serving size:
6 cups	10 minutes plus 2 hours to soak tomatoes	60 minutes	1 cup

Each serving has:			
250 calories	2g total fat	0g saturated fat	0g trans fat
0mg cholesterol	220mg sodium	50g total carbohydrates	10g dietary fiber
7g sugars	12g protein	47mg calcium	3mg iron

5 cups water or vegetable broth

1 cup sun-dried tomatoes

1¼ cups wild rice, rinsed well

1 (15-oz.) can no-salt-added chickpeas, rinsed and drained

1 (14-oz.) can artichoke hearts packed in water, rinsed and drained

1. In a small bowl, combine 2 cups water and sun-dried tomatoes, and set aside to soak for 2 hours. Drain off and discard water.

2. In a medium saucepan over high heat, bring remaining 3 cups water to a boil. Add wild rice, reduce heat to low, and simmer, partially covered, for 45 to 50 minutes or until nearly all liquid is absorbed.

3. Turn off heat and allow rice to stand for 10 minutes or until remaining liquid is absorbed.

4. Stir in sun-dried tomatoes, chickpeas, and artichoke hearts. Serve warm.

PLANT PITFALL

Wild rice needs to be rinsed very well before cooking because it has a tendency to hold on to pebbles, hulls, and dirt. Soak in warm water for a few minutes to allow any debris to be loosened. Then skim off what you can and use a colander or a sifter to wash away the rest.

Collard Greens with Beans and Barley

The delightful blends of textures, sweet and pungent flavors, and bright colors of this staple dish will keep you thinking about seconds.

Yield:	Prep time:	Cook time:	Serving size:
6 cups	10 minutes	10 minutes	1½ cups

Each serving has:			
400 calories	2.5g total fat	0g saturated fat	0g trans fat
0mg cholesterol	570mg sodium	84g total carbohydrates	19g dietary fiber
4g sugars	15g protein	171mg calcium	4mg iron

4½ cups water	3 cups vegetable broth
1 large bunch collard greens, rinsed and chopped	1 (15-oz.) can cannellini beans, rinsed and drained
1 large yellow onion, chopped	¼ tsp. freshly ground black pepper
2 large cloves garlic, minced	4½ cups cooked barley
2 TB. whole-grain oat flour	

1. In a medium pot over medium-high heat, bring 4 cups water to a boil. Add collard greens, and blanch for 1 or 2 minutes or until cooked down and starting to darken in color. Drain.

2. In a separate large pot over medium heat, sauté onion and garlic in remaining ½ cup water for 5 minutes or until onion is translucent.

3. In a medium bowl, whisk together oat flour and vegetable broth, and add to onion mixture. Bring to a boil, and add cannellini beans and black pepper. Reduce heat to low, and simmer, stirring, for 1 minute.

4. Add blanched greens and cooked barley, and simmer, stirring frequently, until flavors are melded and nearly all liquid is absorbed. Serve warm.

 HEALTHY HINT

Blanching is an excellent way to preserve nutrient content and alter the texture of vegetables. When used instead of boiling, baking, or roasting, more of the vitamins, minerals, and phytonutrients remain.

Roasted Cheesy Cauliflower

This may be the simplest dish you've ever made, and yet you won't be able to stop yourself from finishing the whole thing! Think warm and toasty sprinkled with nutty cheese.

Yield:	Prep time:	Cook time:	Serving size:
2 cups	5 minutes	20 to 25 minutes	1 cup

Each serving has:			
84 calories	0.5g total fat	0g saturated fat	0g trans fat
0mg cholesterol	88mg sodium	16g total carbohydrates	8g dietary fiber
7g sugars	8g protein	63mg calcium	1mg iron

1 medium head cauliflower, cut into florets

1 TB. nutritional yeast flakes

1. Preheat the oven to 400°F. Line a baking sheet with a silicone baking mat.

2. Lay cauliflower florets on the baking sheet, and place in the oven. Bake for 20 to 25 minutes or until soft edges are golden brown.

3. Remove from the oven, and sprinkle with nutritional yeast flakes. Serve warm.

Variation: For a richer dish, substitute 2 tablespoons Parmesan Shake (recipe in Chapter 19) for the nutritional yeast flakes.

HEALTHY HINT

Cauliflower provides almost a day's worth of vitamin C and is a member of the extremely health-promoting, cancer-fighting cruciferous vegetable group. Roasting it brings out the subtle sweet flavors and is a truly enjoyable treat.

Beans and Greens Chili

This warm and spicy chili is earthy and fiery and will fill you up no matter how hungry you are.

Yield:	Prep time:	Cook time:	Serving size:
8 cups	10 minutes	50 to 60 minutes	1⅓ cups

Each serving has:			
320 calories	2g total fat	0g saturated fat	0g trans fat
0mg cholesterol	180mg sodium	63g total carbohydrates	21g dietary fiber
13g sugars	18g protein	206mg calcium	5mg iron

1 medium yellow onion, chopped

2 medium carrots, chopped

3 ribs celery, chopped

2 cups vegetable broth

2 (15-oz.) cans kidney beans, drained and rinsed

1 (15-oz.) can chickpeas, drained and rinsed

1 (28-oz.) can chopped tomatoes, with juice

1 (6-oz.) can tomato paste

8 to 12 medium baby bella mushrooms, sliced

1 (15-oz.) can corn, rinsed and drained

2 or 3 TB. chili powder

1 TB. freshly ground black pepper

1 TB. curry powder

4 cups chopped leafy green vegetables

1. In a large soup pot over medium heat, sauté onions, carrots, and celery in ½ cup vegetable broth for 5 minutes or until onions are translucent.

2. Add kidney beans, chickpeas, chopped tomatoes, tomato paste, mushrooms, corn, chili powder, black pepper, curry powder, and remaining 1½ cups vegetable broth. Stir to combine. Reduce heat to medium-low, and simmer for 40 to 50 minutes, stirring occasionally.

3. When chili appears soft, mix in leafy greens and turn off heat. Serve warm.

HEALTHY HINT

Feel free to experiment with different combinations of beans, veggies, and spices in this chili. Use it as a template to highlight your favorites or whatever you have in your cupboard.

Super Snacks

In This Chapter

- Healthful hummus
- Sassy spreads
- Delicious dips

When the snack urge hits, you've come to the right place. The indulgent dips and spreads in this chapter are your ticket to whole-food heaven. Turn these recipes into a meal by spreading them on whole-grain breads, topping your salads with them, or eating enough to make you feel fulfilled.

As you omit all the old-school food rules about how many meals and snacks to eat in a day, you'll tune in to your body's actual needs. Many times, you may notice you only feel like eating something light, while other occasions will call for something more substantial. The light fare in this chapter lends itself to those lighter moods.

However, if you happen to be voraciously hungry, these dishes can be enjoyed as sides, appetizers, or just in larger quantities. One of my favorite mid-day meals is Simply Hummus with corn thins ... but I eat at least half of the whole recipe! Dipping and scooping is fun and satisfying, and this fills me up for hours!

Simply Hummus

This velvety spread delights with lemon accents and garlic undertones.

Yield:	Prep time:	Serving size:	
3 cups	5 minutes	½ cup	
Each serving has:			
150 calories	1g total fat	0g saturated fat	0g trans fat
0mg cholesterol	30mg sodium	26g total carbohydrates	6g dietary fiber
less than 1g sugars	9g protein	63mg calcium	2mg iron

2 (15-oz.) cans chickpeas, rinsed and drained	2 TB. nutritional yeast flakes
¼ cup freshly squeezed lemon juice	½ cup water
2 medium cloves garlic, peeled	¼ tsp. freshly ground black pepper
	¼ tsp. ground paprika

1. In a food processor fitted with an S blade, combine chickpeas, lemon juice, garlic, nutritional yeast flakes, water, black pepper, and paprika. Process for 2 or 3 minutes or until finely ground.

2. Scrape down the sides of the food processor bowl with a wooden spoon, and process for 1 minute longer.

3. Transfer mixture to a serving bowl, and serve with whole-grain crackers or tortillas; with sliced Persian cucumbers, tomatoes, and carrots; or on salad as a dressing, if desired. Store any leftovers in the refrigerator, covered, for up to 4 days.

Variation: For added color, nutrients, and a flavor kick, top with microgreens, sprouts, or shredded leafy greens. Before adding the garlic into the food processor, try roasting it for a smokier flavor. To do this, slice the top off of the entire head and place it on a silicone baking mat– or parchment paper–lined baking sheet. Roast in a 400°F oven for 20 to 25 minutes or until cloves are soft.

HEALTHY HINT

Chickpeas are filled with soluble and insoluble fibers, protein, and a ton of flavor. Making hummus from dried beans is easy and tastes even better than the canned version. Try rinsing and then soaking them for a few hours first. Then rinse again. Finally, cook at a ratio of 3 cups water per 1 cup beans. They become tender after cooking for 1 to 1½ hours.

Indian Hummus

If you like curry, you'll love the unique flavor combination of this hummus. Sweet, strong, and spicy, this hummus can complement less intense items or stand on its own.

Yield:	Prep time:	Serving size:	
2¼ cups	10 minutes	½ cup	
Each serving has:			
250 calories	4.5g total fat	1g saturated fat	0g trans fat
0mg cholesterol	10mg sodium	46g total carbohydrates	8g dietary fiber
20g sugars	9g protein	60mg calcium	3mg iron

2 (15-oz.) cans chickpeas, rinsed and drained	1 tsp. turmeric
	¼ tsp. freshly ground black pepper
2 TB. freshly squeezed lemon juice	2 medium pitted dates or 4 TB. Date Paste
2 medium cloves garlic, minced	(recipe in Chapter 19)
2 TB. cashew butter	½ cup water
1 tsp. *curry powder*	1 cup loosely packed raisins

1. In a food processor fitted with an S blade, combine chickpeas, lemon juice, garlic, cashew butter, curry powder, turmeric, black pepper, dates, and water. Process for 2 or 3 minutes or until finely ground.

2. Scrape down the sides of the food processor bowl with a wooden spoon, and process for 30 more seconds. Sprinkle in raisins, and pulse for 10 seconds or until well combined.

3. Transfer hummus to a serving bowl, and serve with whole-wheat naan bread, whole-grain crackers, or raw vegetables, if desired. Store any leftovers in the refrigerator, covered, for up to 4 days.

Variation: You can use raisins instead of the currants if you like. Natural peanut butter or raw tahini are also good in place of the cashew butter.

DEFINITION

Curry powder is a blend of spices native to India. Although you'll find many different variations, most include turmeric, ginger, paprika, coriander, cumin, pepper, cloves, fenugreek, fennel seeds, curry leaves, and garlic.

Sweet Pea Guacamole

If you love guacamole, you'll delight in this sweeter, milder version. Garlicky and zesty, the sweetness of the peas balances out the flavors.

Yield:	Prep time:	Serving size:	
4 cups	20 minutes	½ cup	
Each serving has:			
180 calories	11g total fat	1.5g saturated fat	0g trans fat
0mg cholesterol	110mg sodium	18g total carbohydrates	8g dietary fiber
1g sugars	6g protein	55mg calcium	2mg iron

3 medium ripe avocados, peeled and pitted

¼ cup freshly squeezed lemon or lime juice

1 tsp. chili powder

½ tsp. freshly ground black pepper

1 cup frozen peas, thawed

1 (15-oz.) can no-salt-added cannellini beans, rinsed and drained

1 or 2 medium cloves garlic, peeled (optional)

½ cup commercially prepared oil-free, low-sodium salsa

1. In a large bowl, mash avocados with a fork until less lumpy. Add lemon juice, chili powder, and black pepper, and smash with the fork until creamy.

2. In a food processor fitted with an S blade or a blender, combine peas, cannellini beans, and garlic (if using). Process or blend for 10 seconds or only until mixed well but still grainy.

3. Add avocado mixture and salsa, and process or blend for 5 to 10 seconds. Scrape down the sides of the food processor bowl with a wooden spoon, and process for 5 to 10 more seconds or just until evenly combined.

4. Transfer to a serving bowl, and serve with homemade chips, corn thins, or whole-grain tortillas; on a baked potato; or in a salad, if desired. Store any leftovers in the refrigerator, covered, for up to 2 days.

Variation: You can also use a commercially prepared guacamole or one from a restaurant if you can't find ripe avocados. Just replace the avocados, lemon juice, chili powder, and black pepper with 1 cup guacamole.

HEALTHY HINT

To peel and pit an avocado easily, slice it open from the stem vertically around the circumference of the fruit. Pry it in half, and pluck out the pit by stabbing it with the end of a sharp knife or scooping it out with a large spoon. Slide a spoon between the flesh and the peel to remove.

Marinara Corn Cakes

This simple snack is tangy and mild. Basil overtones keep your taste buds content.

Yield:	Prep time:	Serving size:	
4 corn cakes	5 minutes	4 corn cakes	
Each serving has:			
200 calories	5g total fat	0.5g saturated fat	0g trans fat
0mg cholesterol	230mg sodium	23g total carbohydrates	5g dietary fiber
2g sugars	12g protein	84mg calcium	2mg iron

¼ cup oil-free marinara sauce, at room temperature or heated

4 corn or rice thins

2 TB. minced fresh basil

3 oz. extra-firm tofu, thinly sliced

1. Spread 1 tablespoon marinara sauce onto each corn thin.

2. Sprinkle ½ tablespoon basil onto each corn thin, and cover with sliced tofu.

Variation: Corn thins are similar to rice cakes, as they're simply puffed corn. You can substitute rice cakes instead or make these on a whole-grain cracker, tortilla, or bread.

HEALTHY HINT

Opt for an oil-free marinara sauce when buying commercial brands. The label should indicate "fat-free" or "oil-free," but to be certain, read the ingredients list.

Savory Nut Spread

Cheesy and pungent, this spread brings out tastes of the Mediterranean, thanks to the sun-dried tomatoes and *tahini*.

Yield:	Prep time:	Serving size:
1½ cups	10 minutes plus 2 hours for soaking	¼ cup

Each serving has:			
160 calories	12g total fat	2g saturated fat	0g trans fat
0mg cholesterol	60mg sodium	10g total carbohydrates	2g dietary fiber
2g sugars	6g protein	13mg calcium	2mg iron

2⅓ cups water

1½ cups raw cashews

4 sun-dried tomatoes

2 TB. nutritional yeast flakes

1 TB. raw tahini

1 TB. freshly squeezed lemon juice

½ tsp. tamari

½ tsp. garlic powder

½ tsp. ground paprika

¼ tsp. freshly ground black pepper (optional)

1. In a small bowl, combine 2 cups water with cashews and sun-dried tomatoes. Set aside to soak for 2 hours. Drain off water and rinse well.

2. In a food processor fitted with an S blade, combine cashews, sun-dried tomatoes, nutritional yeast flakes, tahini, lemon juice, remaining ⅓ cup water, tamari, garlic powder, paprika, and black pepper (if using). Process for 2 or 3 minutes or until smooth.

3. Scrape down the sides of the food processor bowl with a wooden spoon, and process for 10 more seconds or until smooth.

4. Transfer mixture to a serving bowl. Serve on whole-grain crackers, with sliced veggies, or on whole-grain bread as a sandwich spread, if desired. Store any leftovers in the refrigerator, covered, for up to 4 days.

Variation: Try this spread using other nuts, like almonds or walnuts, or a combination of different nuts and seeds like sunflower or hempseeds to measure 1½ cups.

DEFINITION

Tahini is a thick, smooth, Middle Eastern paste made of raw, ground, hulled sesame seeds.

Hot "Cheesy" Vegetable Dip

A perfect party dish, this dip is zesty, spicy, and a rainbow of colors. You'll find excuses to make this flavor-filled bubbling delicacy on normal occasions, too.

Yield:	Prep time:	Cook time:	Serving size:
6 cups	10 minutes	50 minutes	1 cup

Each serving has:			
180 calories	3g total fat	0g saturated fat	0g trans fat
0mg cholesterol	410mg sodium	27g total carbohydrates	15g dietary fiber
3g sugars	15g protein	62mg calcium	2mg iron

1 (14-oz.) pkg. silken tofu

2 (14-oz.) cans artichoke hearts packed in water, rinsed and drained

2 large roasted red peppers packed in water, rinsed and drained

2 cups loosely packed fresh spinach, rinsed and dried

¼ cup freshly squeezed lemon juice

2 medium cloves garlic, peeled

6 TB. nutritional yeast flakes

2 TB. *tamari*

1 TB. chopped fresh or 1 tsp. dried parsley

1 tsp. freshly ground black pepper

½ tsp. cayenne

1. Preheat the oven to 350°F.

2. Crumble tofu into a food processor. Add artichoke hearts, roasted red peppers, spinach, lemon juice, garlic, nutritional yeast flakes, tamari, parsley, black pepper, and cayenne. Process for 45 to 60 seconds or until unified and silky.

3. Pour mixture into an 11×7×2-inch baking dish. Bake, covered, for 30 minutes. Uncover and bake for 20 more minutes or until golden brown.

4. Serve hot with whole-grain crackers, pita bread, and cut vegetables, if desired.

DEFINITION

Tamari is a wheat-free, naturally fermented soybean sauce.

Sensational Sweets

Chapter

23

In This Chapter

- Cookies to satisfy your cravings
- Sweet brownies and breads
- Fantastic fruit desserts

Ahh, dessert. The sweets in this chapter are even more indulgent because they're filled with health-promoting ingredients. Delight in the fact that you can satisfy your sweet tooth with these guilt-free treats.

If you love sweets, you'll be pleasantly amazed at how many decadent desserts can be made using only whole-food sweeteners, dates, fruit purées, and maple syrup. Date paste can easily be made (as seen in Chapter 19), purchased in Middle Eastern markets, or ordered online (see Appendix D). Just be sure no added ingredients are included.

From simple fresh fruit to fancy desserts, whole-food, plant-based will satisfy your sweet tooth more than any refined, processed item will. Reintroduce your taste buds to nature's sweetness, and enjoy the flavors and their accompanying health benefits!

Sweet Cream Dip

Redefine comfort food with this velvety sweet combination.

Yield:	Prep time:	Serving size:	
3 cups	5 minutes	½ cup	
Each serving has:			
190 calories	2g total fat	0g saturated fat	0g trans fat
0mg cholesterol	30mg sodium	35g total carbohydrates	0g dietary fiber
34g sugars	5g protein	216mg calcium	1mg iron

1 (14-oz.) pkg. silken tofu

2 TB. alcohol-free vanilla extract

½ cup Date Paste (recipe in Chapter 19)

1. In a blender or food processor, combine tofu, vanilla extract, and Date Paste, and blend for 45 to 60 seconds or until creamy.

2. Use as a topping for baked goods, as a dip for fresh fruits, or as a yogurt, if desired.

Variation: You can use maple syrup instead of Date Paste in this recipe, but the consistency will be thinner. If you prefer the thickness, decrease the amount of maple syrup to ⅓ cup. Or substitute almond (or other-flavored) extract for a more distinctive flavor.

HEALTHY HINT

Within seconds, you can indulge your senses with this versatile dessert or snack. Treat this recipe as a topping, dip, or yogurt for an irresistible pleasure. It also works with fruits throughout the year. Dip apples and bananas in the winter and peaches and berries in the summer.

Unclassic Oatmeal Raisin Cookies

Light and fluffy, these cookies are maple-rich with raisin accents—a new unclassically classic treat.

Yield:	Prep time:	Cook time:	Serving size:
36 cookies	10 minutes	7 to 10 minutes per batch	2 cookies

Each serving has:			
130 calories	1g total fat	0g saturated fat	0g trans fat
0mg cholesterol	75mg sodium	30g total carbohydrates	1g dietary fiber
22g sugars	1g protein	126mg calcium	1mg iron

1 medium ripe banana, peeled and mashed

1 cup Date Paste (recipe in Chapter 19)

1 TB. alcohol-free vanilla extract

¾ cup oat flour

½ tsp. salt

½ tsp. aluminum-free baking powder

½ tsp. baking soda

2 cups old-fashioned rolled oats

1 cup raisins, packed

1. Preheat the oven to 350°F. Line a baking sheet with a silicone baking mat.

2. In a large bowl, mash banana with a fork. Mix in Date Paste and vanilla extract.

3. Slowly stir oat flour, salt, aluminum-free baking powder, and baking soda into banana mixture. When mixture is smooth, add old-fashioned rolled oats and raisins, and stir until evenly distributed.

4. Scoop dough by tablespoons onto the baking sheet. Bake for 7 to 10 minutes per batch or until edges are golden brown.

5. Cool on a wire rack and serve.

Variation: You can add in 1 cup grain-sweetened chocolate chips, found in health food stores or online (see Appendix D) and/or ½ cup chopped walnuts or pecans for a richer dessert.

HEALTHY HINT

Although famous for their high soluble fiber content, oats are also rich in other nutrients, such as manganese, selenium, phosphorus, thiamin, and magnesium.

Figamajigs

This recipe takes fig bars to a whole new level! Hard to believe raw nuts and dried fruits can combine to create such sweet and chewy goodness.

Yield:	Prep time:	Serving size:	
12 bars	5 minutes	1 bar	
Each serving has:			
220 calories	13g total fat	<1g saturated fat	0g trans fat
0mg cholesterol	2mg sodium	26g total carbohydrates	6g dietary fiber
19g sugars	6g protein	34mg calcium	0.5mg iron

2 cups raw almonds	1 cup dried figs
1 cup pitted dates	1 TB. alcohol-free vanilla extract

1. In a food processor fitted with an S blade, process almonds for approximately 30 to 45 seconds or until they form a flourlike consistency.

2. Add dates and figs, and process until mixture begins to clump together.

3. Add vanilla extract, and process for 10 more seconds or until well-combined.

4. Spoon mixture into a 8×8-inch silicone baking pan and press down with your hands. Cut into 12 bars, and serve.

Variation: You can also roll the mixture into balls instead of bars or shape them with cookie cutters to make them fun for kids.

MIXED GREENS

Save beaucoup bucks by using these Figamajigs as energy bars. They cost a fraction of the price when compared to commercial bars. Plus, these have no preservatives or isolated, concentrated vitamins or minerals. Just deliciously *au natural!*

AJ's Peanut Bites

Peanuty and chewy, these are quick treats you'll be making for your friends.

Yield:	Prep time:	Serving size:	
20 bites	5 minutes	1 bite	
Each serving has:			
130 calories	7g total fat	1g saturated fat	0g trans fat
0mg cholesterol	0mg sodium	14g total carbohydrates	2g dietary fiber
10g sugars	4g protein	14mg calcium	0mg iron

2 cups unsalted, roasted peanuts

2 cups pitted dates

1 TB. alcohol-free vanilla extract

1. In a food processor fitted with an S blade, process peanuts for 60 seconds or until a flourlike consistency forms. Don't overprocess, or you'll end up with peanut butter.

2. Slowly add dates, a few at a time, until mixture clumps together. Stop the food processor; if you can easily roll a ball from the mixture in your hands and it sticks, you don't need to add any more dates.

3. Add vanilla extract, and process for 10 more seconds or until well combined.

4. Using your hands, roll mixture into 20 balls, and place on a flat surface. Serve.

Variation: To make **Brownie Bites,** use the same technique, but use these ingredients instead: 2 cups raw walnuts, 2 cups pitted dates, ½ cup cocoa powder, and 1 tablespoon alcohol-free vanilla extract. Add cocoa powder with nuts at the beginning. To make either of these bite variations fancier, you can roll the balls in raw cocoa or carob powder, crushed nuts, or shredded coconut.

HEALTHY HINT

Take these bites as a fresh and homemade on-the-go snack. Treat them like you would a nutrition bar.

Chef AJ's Outrageous Brownies

Indulge your sweet tooth while still eating nutrient-dense. These rich, chocolaty treats will shock your family and friends when they find out how healthful they are. Just be sure you tell them *after* they taste them!

Yield:	Prep time:	Cook time:	Serving size:
16 brownies	10 minutes	30 to 35 minutes	1 brownie

Each serving has:			
240 calories	5g total fat	1.5g saturated fat	0g trans fat
0mg cholesterol	40mg sodium	44g total carbohydrates	3g dietary fiber
33g sugars	3g protein	264mg calcium	2mg iron

1 (15-oz.) can no-salt-added black beans, rinsed and drained

1¼ cups Date Paste (recipe in Chapter 19)

2 TB. ground flaxseeds

1 TB. alcohol-free vanilla extract

½ tsp. caramel extract (optional)

1 tsp. aluminum-free baking powder

½ tsp. baking soda

½ cup alkali-free cocoa powder

¾ cup barley flour

1 cup nondairy, grain-sweetened chocolate chips

½ cup finely chopped raw, unsalted pecans

1. Preheat the oven to 350°F.

2. In a food processor fitted with an S blade, combine black beans and Date Paste, and process for 45 seconds or until smooth.

3. Add flaxseeds, vanilla extract, caramel extract (if using), aluminum-free baking powder, baking soda, and cocoa powder. Process for 30 more seconds. Add barley flour, and process for 5 to 10 more seconds or just until combined. Stir in chocolate chips.

4. Pour batter into an 8×8-inch silicone baking pan. Sprinkle pecans on top. Bake for 30 to 35 minutes or until middle does not jiggle and a toothpick inserted comes out clean. Cool on a wire rack for 20 minutes before serving.

Variation: You can use 1¼ cups maple syrup instead of the Date Paste and also substitute ½ cup hempseeds for the pecans. A few extra chocolate chips sprinkled on top add visual and textural appeal.

MIXED GREENS

Caramel extract is a specialty item that's not readily available on your local grocer's shelf. If you can't find it, try other extracts like mint, almond, or lemon in the same quantity to vary the flavor.

Fruity Nut Balls

Take these tangy, tart, sweet, and crunchy portable treats with you wherever you go.

Yield:	Prep time:	Serving size:
14 balls	10 minutes	1 ball

Each serving has:			
160 calories	7g total fat	1g saturated fat	0g trans fat
0mg cholesterol	1mg sodium	21g total carbohydrates	2g dietary fiber
14g sugars	4g protein	23mg calcium	1mg iron

2 cups raw cashews	1 cup dried unsweetened cherries
1 cup pitted dates	1 TB. alcohol-free vanilla extract

1. In a food processor fitted with an S blade, process cashews for approximately 30 to 45 seconds or until they form a flourlike consistency.

2. Add dates and cherries, and process for 2 to 4 minutes or until mixture begins to clump together.

3. Slowly drizzle vanilla extract into mixture, and process for 10 more seconds.

4. Using your hands, roll dough into balls, and serve. Keep covered in the refrigerator for 4 or 5 days.

Variation: Use the same amount of raw peanuts instead of cashews for **Peanut Butter and Jelly Balls.**

PLANT PITFALL

Beware of sugar and oil in dried fruits. Look for unsweetened versions, and be sure the only ingredient listed is the fruit itself.

Chocolate-Chip Pumpkin Bread

This spicy, fudgy bread will tantalize your taste buds. A mix between a pudding and a cake, it's the perfect item to bring to parties … or just keep to yourself at home!

Yield:	Prep time:	Cook time:	Serving size:
1 (9×5-inch) loaf	15 minutes	1 hour	1 slice (5¼×1¾×¾-inch)

Each serving has:			
312 calories	6g total fat	2.5g saturated fat	0g trans fat
0mg cholesterol	160mg sodium	62g total carbohydrates	4g dietary fiber
45g sugars	3g protein	258mg calcium	1mg iron

1 cup Date Paste (recipe in Chapter 19)	½ tsp. baking soda
1 (15-oz.) can pumpkin purée	½ tsp. salt
3 TB. flax eggs (see instructions in Chapter 18)	1 tsp. ground cinnamon
½ cup pure maple syrup	¼ tsp. ground cloves
1 TB. alcohol-free vanilla extract	¼ tsp. ground nutmeg
1½ cups oat flour	¼ tsp. ground ginger
½ tsp. aluminum-free baking powder	1½ cups grain-sweetened chocolate chips

1. Preheat the oven to 350°F.

2. In a large bowl, combine Date Paste, pumpkin purée, flax eggs, maple syrup, and vanilla extract until smooth.

3. Gently stir in oat flour, aluminum-free baking powder, baking soda, salt, cinnamon, cloves, nutmeg, and ginger. Mix until no lumps remain. Add chocolate chips, and evenly distribute throughout.

4. Pour batter into a 9×5-inch loaf pan, and bake for 1 hour. Allow bread to cool before cutting and serving.

PLANT PITFALL

Grain-sweetened chocolate chips are not technically a whole food, and they're a specialty item. But if you can find them, feel comfortable using them in baked goods because the ingredients are completely plant-based as well as sugar- and oil-free. You can also opt for raisins or other dried fruits in place of the chocolate chips.

Dried Fruit Compote

Stewing or simmering dried fruits is a great way to re-hydrate them as well as infuse them with extra flavor. This warm fruit compote makes it easy to get your servings of fruit during the cold winter months in a sweet and spicy way.

Yield:	Prep time:	Cook time:	Serving size:
5 cups	5 to 10 minutes	10 to 12 minutes	1¼ cups

Each serving has:			
441 calories	1g total fat	0g saturated fat	0g trans fat
0mg cholesterol	10mg sodium	113g total carbohydrates	13g dietary fiber
83g sugars	5g protein	104mg calcium	4mg iron

1½ cups dried peaches or other large dried fruit, cut in half

⅔ cup dried figs, cut in half

⅔ cup dried prunes, pitted and cut in half

⅔ cup dried dates, pitted and cut in half

⅓ cup raisins

⅓ cup dried cranberries or cherries

1 large orange

1½ cups water

1 (3-in.) cinnamon stick

1 (½-in.) slice fresh ginger

1. In a medium saucepan, combine peaches, figs, prunes, and dates. Add raisins and cranberries.

2. Using a vegetable peeler, remove long strips of peel from orange and then juice orange using a reamer or juicer. Add orange peel and orange juice to the saucepan, along with water, cinnamon stick, and ginger.

3. Place the saucepan over medium heat, and cook for 10 to 12 minutes or until dried fruit is plump and soft. Remove from heat. Remove cinnamon stick and ginger slice, and discard. Serve warm or cold as desired.

Variation: Individual servings can also be topped with soy yogurt and chopped nuts, if desired. You can also replace ½ cup water with apple juice, white grape juice, or white wine, and serve the compote as a dessert with slices of cake or scoops of nondairy ice cream or sorbet.

PLANT PITFALL

Choose untreated organic dried fruits over those that have been treated with sulfur dioxide, a controversial preservative often used to prevent discoloration of foods due to oxidation.

Baked Apples

An old-time fall dessert, these apples are filled with the flavor of sweetly spiced nuts and dried fruits.

Yield:	Prep time:	Cook time:	Serving size:
6 apples	10 to 12 minutes	35 to 45 minutes	1 apple

Each serving has:			
225 calories	4g total fat	0g saturated fat	0g trans fat
0mg cholesterol	6mg sodium	51g total carbohydrates	6g dietary fiber
40g sugars	2g protein	28mg calcium	1mg iron

½ cup apple juice	3 TB. dried cranberries
4 TB. maple syrup	1 TB. minced fresh ginger
¼ cup coarsely chopped raw walnuts	½ tsp. ground cinnamon
3 TB. raisins	6 large Gala or other apples, cut in half and cored

1. Preheat the oven to 375°F.

2. Pour apple juice and 2 tablespoons maple syrup into a 9×13-inch silicone baking pan, and stir well to combine. Set aside.

3. In a small bowl, combine walnuts, remaining 2 tablespoons maple syrup, raisins, dried cranberries, ginger, and cinnamon, and stir well.

4. Fill cavity of each apple with walnut mixture, and place filled apples into the baking pan.

5. Bake for 35 to 45 minutes or until apples are tender but not mushy, basting apples with pan juices every 15 minutes during baking. Remove from the oven.

6. Serve apples with pan juices spooned over the top. For an extra special treat, serve with scoops of nondairy ice cream or sorbet, if desired.

Variations: Replace walnuts with almonds or sunflower seeds and dried cranberries with chopped dates, apricots, or other dried fruits. For **Baked Pears,** cut pears in half lengthwise and remove their cores, fill cavities, and bake them open faced.

HEALTHY HINT

Silicone bakeware is a safe way to bake without oil. Nothing sticks to its surface and because it's an inert chemical, it's safe to use. Plus, it's made in many shapes and sizes to accommodate any recipe. Just be sure not to use it on direct heat sources to prevent melting.

activities of daily living (ADL)   Self-care skills necessary for day-to-day function, including walking, sitting up, preparing meals, eating, lifting, and bending.

adaptation   Your body's physiologic response to exercise. It occurs with a persistent training regimen and means your body has learned to cope with the stress you've placed on it from your current program. To avoid plateaus, you have to change your workout frequently.

agar agar   A gelatinous substance derived from seaweed that works as a thickening agent and can replace gelatin as a plant-based substitute.

allspice   Named for its flavor echoes of several spices (cinnamon, cloves, nutmeg), allspice is used in many desserts and in rich marinades and stews.

almonds   Mild, sweet, and crunchy nuts that combine nicely with creamy and sweet food items.

artichoke hearts   The center part of the artichoke flower, often found canned in grocery stores.

arugula   A spicy-peppery garden plant with leaves that resemble a dandelion and have a distinctive—and very sharp—flavor.

atherosclerosis   The process of hardening and thickening of the arterial walls, associated with an increased risk for heart attacks, strokes, and other vascular diseases.

atherosclerotic plaque   A build-up of cholesterol, calcium, cellular debris, and fatty materials in the walls of the blood vessels as a consequence of atherosclerosis.

atrophic gastritis   A chronic inflammation of the stomach lining that interferes with vitamin B_{12} absorption. This condition affects up to half of adults over age 60.

autoimmune disease   An illness caused by the body attacking itself. This includes illnesses such as type 1 diabetes, multiple sclerosis, rheumatoid arthritis, and lupus.

balsamic vinegar   Vinegar produced primarily in Italy from a specific type of grape and aged in wood barrels. It's heavier, darker, and sweeter than most vinegars.

basal metabolic rate (BMR)   A measure of the rate of metabolism, it's the energy needed to sustain the metabolic activities of cells and tissues to maintain circulatory, respiratory, gastrointestinal, and renal processes.

basil   A flavorful, almost sweet, resinous herb delicious with tomatoes and used in all kinds of Italian or Mediterranean-style dishes.

beriberi   A thiamin deficiency resulting in difficulty walking; loss of sensation or function in the legs, hands, or feet; tingling; and mental confusion.

black pepper   A biting and pungent seasoning, freshly ground pepper is a must for many dishes and adds an extra level of flavor and taste.

blanch   To place a food in boiling water for about 1 minute (or less) to partially cook the exterior and then submerge in or rinse with cool water to halt the cooking.

bone mineral density (BMD)   The amount of minerals in any volume of bone.

calisthenics   A form of exercise intended to develop strength and flexibility using resistance provided by your body and minimal or no equipment.

carbohydrate   A nutritional component found in starches, sugars, fruits, and vegetables that causes a rise in blood glucose levels. Carbohydrates supply energy and many important nutrients, including vitamins, minerals, and antioxidants.

carcinogens   Agents or substances that cause or exacerbate cancer growth.

cardiac output   The total amount of blood flow from the heart during a specified period of time, or stroke volume multiplied by heart rate. Cardiac output is regulated by the amount of nutrients and oxygen required by the cells as well as the requirement to remove wastes.

cayenne   A fiery spice made from (hot) chile peppers, especially the cayenne chile, a slender, red, and very hot pepper.

certified organic   A labeling term that means a food or food product has been produced following the guidelines of the USDA National Organic Standards Board. Organic production is a system that integrates cultural, biological, and mechanical practices that foster cycling of resources, promote ecological balance, and conserve biodiversity.

chickpeas (or **garbanzo beans**)   Yellow-gold, roundish beans used as the base ingredient in hummus. Chickpeas are high in fiber and low in fat.

chili powder   A seasoning blend that includes chile pepper, cumin, garlic, and oregano. Proportions vary among different versions, but they all offer a warm, rich flavor.

Chinese five-spice powder   A seasoning blend of cinnamon, anise, ginger, fennel, and pepper.

chop   To cut into pieces, usually qualified by an adverb such as "*coarsely* chopped" or by a size measurement such as "chopped into ½-inch pieces." "Finely chopped" is much closer to *mince*.

cilantro   A member of the parsley family used in Mexican cooking (especially salsa) and some Asian dishes. Use in moderation, as the flavor can overwhelm. The seed of the cilantro is the spice coriander.

cinnamon   A rich, aromatic spice commonly used in baking or desserts. Cinnamon can also be used for delicious and interesting entrées.

circulatory system   The heart, arteries, capillaries, and veins. This system is responsible for transporting blood, oxygen, and nutrients to all cells in the body.

coconut water   The clear liquid found inside a young coconut, which is extremely high in electrolytes and makes an excellent natural sports drink.

coenzymes   Small, nonprotein molecules that enhance the action of an enzyme.

core   The group of muscles located around the trunk of the body. Typically, this includes the abdominal muscles (rectus abdominis, transverse abdominis, external and internal obliques), pelvic floor muscles, and spinal stabilizer muscles.

coriander   A rich, warm, spicy seed used in all types of recipes, from African to South American, from entrées to desserts.

cumin   A fiery, smoky-tasting spice popular in Middle Eastern and Indian dishes. Cumin is a seed; ground cumin seed is the most common form used in cooking.

curry   Rich, spicy, Indian-style sauces and the dishes prepared with them. A curry uses curry powder as its base seasoning.

curry powder   A ground blend of rich and flavorful spices used as a basis for curry and many other Indian-influenced dishes. Common ingredients include hot pepper, nutmeg, cumin, cinnamon, pepper, and turmeric. Some curry can also be found in paste form.

detoxification   The process of cleansing and removing toxic compounds that may have accumulated in the organs over a period of time.

diabetic ketoacidosis   A life-threatening situation caused by insufficient insulin, leading to high blood sugar levels, nausea, vomiting, abdominal pain, dehydration, ketones in the urine, acidosis, and the potential for coma and death.

dietary cholesterol   A waxy steroid metabolite found in cell membranes and transported via the blood of all animals. An essential structural component of cell membranes, cholesterol is necessary for the manufacture of bile acids, steroid hormones, and fat-soluble vitamins, including vitamins A, D, E, and K.

diverticulosis   A condition in which the colon has small outpouchings that may lead to inflammation (diverticulitis).

DNA   An acronym for deoxyribonucleic acid, this nucleic acid (one of two, with the other being RNA) is found in the nucleus of every cell in the body and contains the genetic instructions for the development and function for all life forms.

electrolytes   Minerals found in the blood that help balance fluids and maintain normal functions, like your heart's rhythm and muscle contraction. The main electrolytes are sodium, potassium, chloride, magnesium, calcium, phosphate, and bicarbonate.

endorphins   Neurochemicals produced in the body that act as natural painkillers.

energy density   The number of calories per gram of food (kcal/g).

excitotoxins   Toxic molecules, like MSG or aspartame, that stimulate nerve cells so much they're damaged or killed.

flexibility   A joint's ability to move freely through a full and normal range of motion. Many factors influence joint mobility, including genetics, the joint structure itself, neuromuscular coordination, and strength of the opposing muscle group.

flexitarian   A contraction of "flexible vegetarian," or someone who eats mostly plant-based foods but occasionally eats meat, poultry, or fish.

free radicals   High-energy particles with at least one unpaired electron that go wild in the body, ricocheting around trying to match up their unpaired electrons. This causes damage and leads to heart disease, cancers, autoimmune disease, macular degeneration, impaired immunity, and accelerated aging.

garlic   A member of the onion family. A pungent and flavorful element in many savory dishes. A garlic bulb contains multiple cloves. Each clove, when chopped, provides about 1 teaspoon garlic. Most recipes call for cloves or chopped garlic by the teaspoon.

gastric distention   A swelling or bloating of the stomach.

gestational diabetes (GDM)   Any degree of glucose intolerance that's first discovered during pregnancy. Although the condition usually resolves after delivery, it increases long-term risk of developing type 2 diabetes. Children of moms with GDM are at increased risk of obesity, glucose intolerance, and diabetes in late adolescence and young adulthood. GDM complicates approximately 7 percent of pregnancies, according to the American Diabetes Association.

ginger   Available in fresh root or dried, ground form, ginger adds a pungent, sweet, and spicy quality to a dish.

glomerular filtration rate (GFR)   A measure of kidney function equal to the rate at which fluid filters through the kidneys.

goiter   An abnormally enlarged thyroid gland most commonly due to iodine deficiency in the diet but that can also occur with other thyroid disease.

gomashio   A Japanese condiment comprised of a blend of toasted sesame seeds, salt, and sometimes sea vegetables.

GRAS   An acronym for the phrase "generally recognized as safe." Under the Food and Drug Administration's Federal Food, Drug, and Cosmetic Act, "any substance that is intentionally added to food is considered a food additive, that is subject to premarket review and approval by FDA, unless the substance is generally recognized, among qualified experts, as having been adequately shown to be safe under the conditions of its intended use, or unless the use of the substance is otherwise excluded from the definition of a food additive."

hemorrhoids   Dilated veins in the anus or rectum typically caused by constipation or strains due to diarrhea or pregnancy.

herbes de Provence   A seasoning mix including basil, fennel, marjoram, rosemary, sage, and thyme, common in the south of France.

herbivores   Plant-eaters.

herbs   Plants valued for their aromas, flavors, or medicinal qualities.

hyponatremia   An abnormally low concentration of sodium (less than 130 mEq per liter) in the blood that can cause cells to malfunction and can be fatal. Hyponatremia has become common in high-endurance events because it can result from prolonged, heavy sweating with failure to replenish sodium or from excessive water consumption.

insoluble fiber   Fiber that's not soluble in water and consists mainly of lignin, cellulose, and hemicelluloses. This type of fiber is primarily found in the bran layers of cereal grains.

insulin shock   A condition that occurs when too much insulin is in the blood, leading to severely low blood sugar (hypoglycemia) and possibly resulting in convulsions and coma.

iodine   A trace mineral required from the diet to help with metabolism.

julienne   A French word meaning "to slice into very thin pieces."

lacto-ovo vegetarians   Vegetarians who consume dairy products and eggs.

lactose intolerance   The inability to digest lactose, the sugar component of milk, due to the body's failure to produce the enzyme lactase. Gastrointestinal symptoms vary from mild to extreme and can include gas, bloating, cramps, diarrhea, and extreme pain.

lentils   Tiny lens-shape pulses used in European, Middle Eastern, and Indian cuisines.

lymphatic system   Includes vessels and lymph nodes separate from the circulatory system that filter out microorganisms and other toxins before returning fluid and protein to the blood. It carries white blood cells throughout the body to help fight infection.

macrominerals   Also considered "bulk elements." Your body requires these minerals in amounts of 100mg per day or greater.

marjoram   A sweet herb, a cousin of and similar to oregano, popular in Greek, Spanish, and Italian dishes.

meat analogues   Products intended to imitate the texture, flavor, and appearance of meats and that are made from non-animal-based ingredients.

metabolic syndrome   A cluster of conditions, including obesity, high cholesterol, hypertension, and high blood sugar, that lead to vascular and other chronic diseases.

metabolism   The whole range of biochemical processes that occur in the body and are necessary for the maintenance of life.

microminerals   Also known as "trace elements," these are present in minute amounts in the body's tissues and are essential in much smaller quantities (closer to 15mg per day or less) for optimal health, growth, and development.

miso   A fermented, flavorful soybean paste that is key in many Japanese dishes.

neuropathy   Damage to the nerves that causes tingling, weakness, pain, and/or numbness, usually in the legs, feet, toes, arms, and fingers.

nori   The Japanese name for seaweed; typically dried, toasted, made into flat sheets, and used for sushi as a wrapper.

norito   A combination of *nori* and *burrito*, these rolls, filled with crunchy and savory filling and wrapped in crispy nori sheets, ultimately end up looking, and being eaten, like burritos.

omnivore   A person or animal who eats anything.

osteopenia   A condition in which bone mineral density appears to be lower than normal. It's considered a precursor to osteoporosis.

oxalates   Compounds found in plant foods (especially leafy greens) that greatly reduce the body's absorption of calcium, iron, and magnesium. Some of these oxalates can be broken down by soaking or cooking. A build-up of oxalates in the body can potentially cause kidney stones.

oxidation   The browning of fruit flesh that happens over time and with exposure to air. Minimize oxidation by rubbing the cut surfaces with a lemon half. Oxidation also affects wine, which is why the taste changes over time after a bottle is opened.

passive immunity   The temporary protection against disease from the already-made antibodies of one human given to another.

pellagra   Illness caused by a deficiency in niacin resulting in scaly skin sores, delusions, diarrhea, inflamed mucous membranes, and mental confusion.

Persian cucumbers   Mini seedless cucumbers that are crisp, refreshing, and available throughout the year.

phytoestrogens   Plant compounds, similar to the hormone estrogen, that look and act like estrogen in the body.

plant-based milks   Beverages made from soy, almonds, rice, hemp, and oats fortified with calcium, vitamin B_{12}, and vitamin D that can be used in the same fashion as cow's milk but without the health risks.

prebiotics   Fermentable carbohydrates that encourage the growth of friendly bacteria in the GI tract. These friendly bacteria and their by-products inhibit the growth of harmful bacteria and yeasts, reduce cancer-promoting compounds, improve absorption of minerals, and perhaps reduce food intolerances and allergies.

protein combining   A practice taught by nutrition experts to ensure people consumed adequate amounts of all the essential amino acids. Certain foods were recommended to be eaten together at the same meal (grains and legumes, for example) to prevent protein deficiency. This method is antiquated because it has been confirmed that the body can make proteins out of pooled amino acids as long as a variety of plant foods is consumed and energy needs are met.

purines   A class of aromatic organic compounds that are components of nucleic acids (DNA and RNA) found in human and animal tissue.

refined foods   Foods stripped of their intact parts, as when whole grains have their bran and/or germ removed (leaving only the endosperm); examples include white flour and white rice. Refined products can also be called "polished" or "processed."

resting heart rate   The number of times the heart beats when you are completely inactive.

retinopathy   A disease of the small blood vessels in the retina of the eyes that can eventually result in impaired vision and blindness.

rice vinegar   Vinegar produced from fermented rice or rice wine, popular in Asian-style dishes. Different from rice wine vinegar.

sage   An herb with a musty yet fruity lemon-rind scent and "sunny" flavor.

salsa   A style of mixing fresh vegetables and/or fresh fruit in a coarse chop. Salsa can be spicy or not, fruit-based or not, and served as a starter on its own (with chips, for example) or as a companion to a main course.

satiety   The state of fullness and satisfaction after eating adequately.

sauté   To pan-cook over lower heat than used for frying.

scurvy   A disorder caused by vitamin C deficiency characterized by spongy gums, bleeding of the skin and gums, and loosening of the teeth.

semi-vegetarian   Someone who excludes some meat, usually red meat, from the diet while still consuming limited amounts of poultry, fish, and/or seafood.

simmer   To boil gently so the liquid barely bubbles.

soluble fiber   The water-soluble form of dietary fiber that has an affinity for water, either dissolving or swelling to form a gel. Soluble fiber is primarily found in fruits, vegetables, oats, barley, legumes, and seaweed.

spices   Any of a variety of dried seeds, roots, barks, fruits, or leaves used to add flavors, colors, or antimicrobial properties to foods.

statistical significance   A measure of how unlikely it is that a result of a study has occurred by chance.

steam   To suspend a food over boiling water and allow the heat of the steam (water vapor) to cook the food. A quick cooking method, steaming preserves the flavor and texture of a food.

stir-fry   To cook small pieces of food in a wok or skillet over high heat, moving and turning the food quickly to cook all sides.

stress hormones   Substances such as cortisol, adrenaline, norepinephrine, and epinephrine secreted by the endocrine system when tension is induced.

stroke volume   The amount of blood pumped from the left ventricle of the heart with one contraction.

supergrains   A term used to represent grains extremely high in essential amino acids, including lysine and methionine, not common in other grains. They're also exceptionally high in fiber, vitamins, and minerals.

synergy   The effect of two or more units working together to produce a result not obtainable by each of the units independently.

tahini   A thick, smooth Middle Eastern paste made of raw, ground, hulled sesame seeds.

tamari   A wheat-free, naturally fermented soybean sauce.

tempeh   An Indonesian food made by culturing and fermenting soybeans into a cake, sometimes mixed with grains or vegetables, and high in protein and fiber.

thermic effect of food (TEF)   The increase in energy expenditure associated with the processes of digestion, absorption, and the metabolism of food.

tofu   A cheeselike substance made from soybeans and soy milk that is high in protein, omega-3 fatty acids, and calcium.

turmeric   A spicy, pungent yellow root used in many dishes, especially Indian cuisine, for color and flavor. Turmeric is the source of the yellow color in many prepared mustards.

umami   A flavor common in Eastern cooking that provides a meaty or savory type of taste. It's considered the fifth flavor after sweet, salty, sour, and bitter.

vegan   A strict vegetarian who avoids consumption and use of all animal products, including animal flesh, dairy, eggs, honey, leather, fur, silk, wool, and pearls.

vegetarians   People who avoid consuming meat, poultry, and fish.

villi   Tiny, fingerlike protrusions that line the small intestines and allow absorption of nutrients from the intestines into the bloodstream.

whole grains   Grains derived from the seeds of grasses, including rice, oats, rye, wheat, wild rice, quinoa, barley, buckwheat, bulgur, corn, millet, amaranth, and sorghum.

whole-food, plant-based diet   A way of eating that emphasizes whole, plant-based foods, including vegetables, fruits, whole grains, and legumes, while avoiding animal products and highly processed foods.

wild rice   Actually a grass with a rich, nutty flavor, popular as an unusual and nutritious side dish.

zest   Small slivers of peel, usually from a citrus fruit such as lemon, lime, or orange.

zester   A kitchen tool used to scrape zest off a fruit. A small grater also works well.

Sample Meal Plans

Although there's no rhyme or reason to what you should eat or when, this meal plan can help you get started. Mix and match however you please, or based on what's in your kitchen at the time. Just eat whole plants and all will be well!

Day 1

Breakfast: It's Easy Being Green Smoothie (Chapter 20)

Lunch: Japanese Noritos (Chapter 20)

Snack: Simply Hummus (Chapter 22) with baby carrots and cucumbers

Dinner: Baked Lentils and Rice Casserole (Chapter 21)

Day 2

Breakfast: Blueberry Banana Pancakes (Chapter 20)

Lunch: Zel's Zesty Rainbow Salad (Chapter 20)

Snack: Sweet Pea Guacamole (Chapter 22) with whole-grain baked corn chips

Dinner: Japanoodles (Chapter 21)

Day 3

Breakfast: Chocolate Almond Butter in a Cup (Chapter 20)

Lunch: Wacky Wild Rice (Chapter 21)

Snack: Sweet Cream Dip (Chapter 23) with apple and banana slices

Dinner: Beans and Greens Chili (Chapter 21)

Day 4

Breakfast: Veggie Tofu Scramble (Chapter 20)

Lunch: Sushi Salad with Creamy Miso Dressing (Chapter 20)

Snack: Savory Nut Spread (Chapter 22) on whole-grain crackers

Dinner: Fiesta Fantastica (Chapter 21)

Day 5

Breakfast: Breakfast Rice Pudding (Chapter 20)

Lunch: Cold Melon Soup (Chapter 20)

Snack: Indian Hummus (Chapter 22) with whole-wheat naan

Dinner: Easy Beans and Quinoa (Chapter 21)

Day 6

Breakfast: Oatmeal with walnuts and berries

Lunch: Cream of Carrot Soup (Chapter 20)

Snack: Unclassic Oatmeal Raisin Cookies (Chapter 23)

Dinner: Herbed Balsamic Pasta (Chapter 21)

Day 7

Breakfast: Mint Chocolate Nib Smoothie (Chapter 20)

Lunch: Mexican Noritos (Chapter 20)

Snack: Hot "Cheesy" Vegetable Dip (Chapter 22)

Dinner: Tempeh stir-fried with vegetables and brown rice

Nutrition Charts

As you've gathered by now, nutrition is pretty important stuff. To help you determine how much of what nutrients you need on a daily basis, check out the following Dietary Reference Intakes, created by the Institute of Medicine's Food and Nutrition Board.

Dietary Reference Intakes (DRIs): Recommended Intakes for Individuals, Vitamins

Food and Nutrition Board, Institute of Medicine, National Academies

Life Stage Group	Vit A (µg/d)[a]	Vit C (mg/d)	Vit D (µg/d)[b,c]	Vit E (mg/d)[d]	Vit K (µg/d)	Thiamin (mg/d)	Riboflavin (mg/d)	Niacin (mg/d)[e]	Vit B6 (mg/d)	Folate (µg/d)[f]	Vit B12 (µg/d)	Pantothenic Acid (mg/d)	Biotin (µg/d)	Choline[g] (mg/d)
Infants														
0–6 mo	400*	40*	5*	4*	2.0*	0.2*	0.3*	2*	0.1*	65*	0.4*	1.7*	5*	125*
7–12 mo	500*	50*	5*	5*	2.5*	0.3*	0.4*	4*	0.3*	80*	0.5*	1.8*	6*	150*
Children														
1–3 y	300	15	5*	6	30*	0.5	0.5	6	0.5	150	0.9	2*	8*	200*
4–8 y	400	25	5*	7	55*	0.6	0.6	8	0.6	200	1.2	3*	12*	250*
Males														
9–13 y	600	45	5*	11	60*	0.9	0.9	12	1.0	300	1.8	4*	20*	375*
14–18 y	900	75	5*	15	75*	1.2	1.3	16	1.3	400	2.4	5*	25*	550*
19–30 y	900	90	5*	15	120*	1.2	1.3	16	1.3	400	2.4	5*	30*	550*
31–50 y	900	90	5*	15	120*	1.2	1.3	16	1.3	400	2.4	5*	30*	550*
51–70 y	900	90	10*	15	120*	1.2	1.3	16	1.7	400	2.4	5*	30*	550*
> 70 y	900	90	15*	15	120*	1.2	1.3	16	1.7	400	2.4	5*	30*	550*
Females														
9–13 y	600	45	5*	11	60*	0.9	0.9	12	1.0	300	1.8	4*	20*	375*
14–18 y	700	65	5*	15	75*	1.0	1.0	14	1.2	400[i]	2.4	5*	25*	400*
19–30 y	700	75	5*	15	90*	1.1	1.1	14	1.3	400[i]	2.4	5*	30*	425*
31–50 y	700	75	5*	15	90*	1.1	1.1	14	1.3	400[i]	2.4	5*	30*	425*
51–70 y	700	75	10*	15	90*	1.1	1.1	14	1.5	400	2.4[h]	5*	30*	425*
> 70 y	700	75	15*	15	90*	1.1	1.1	14	1.5	400	2.4[h]	5*	30*	425*
Pregnancy														
14–18 y	750	80	5*	15	75*	1.4	1.4	18	1.9	600[j]	2.6	6*	30*	450*
19–30 y	770	85	5*	15	90*	1.4	1.4	18	1.9	600[j]	2.6	6*	30*	450*
31–50 y	770	85	5*	15	90*	1.4	1.4	18	1.9	600[j]	2.6	6*	30*	450*
Lactation														
14–18 y	1,200	115	5*	19	75*	1.4	1.6	17	2.0	500	2.8	7*	35*	550*
19–30 y	1,300	120	5*	19	90*	1.4	1.6	17	2.0	500	2.8	7*	35*	550*
31–50 y	1,300	120	5*	19	90*	1.4	1.6	17	2.0	500	2.8	7*	35*	550*

NOTE: This table (taken from the DRI reports, see www.nap.edu) presents Recommended Dietary Allowances (RDAs) in **bold type** and Adequate Intakes (AIs) in ordinary type followed by an asterisk (*). RDAs and AIs may both be used as goals for individual intake. RDAs are set to meet the needs of almost all (97 to 98 percent) individuals in a group. For healthy breastfed infants, the AI is the mean intake. The AI for other life stage and gender groups is believed to cover needs of all individuals in the group, but lack of data or uncertainty in the data prevent being able to specify with confidence the percentage of individuals covered by this intake.

[a] As retinol activity equivalents (RAEs). 1 RAE = 1 µg retinol, 12 µg β-carotene, 24 µg α-carotene, or 24 µg β-cryptoxanthin. The RAE for dietary provitamin A carotenoids is twofold greater than retinol equivalents (RE), whereas the RAE for preformed vitamin A is the same as RE.

[b] As cholecalciferol. 1 µg cholecalciferol = 40 IU vitamin D.

[c] In the absence of adequate exposure to sunlight.

[d] As α-tocopherol. α-Tocopherol includes *RRR*-α-tocopherol, the only form of α-tocopherol that occurs naturally in foods, and the 2*R*-stereoisomeric forms of α-tocopherol (*RRR-*, *RSR-*, *RRS-*, and *RSS*-α-tocopherol) that occur in fortified foods and supplements. It does not include the 2*S*-stereoisomeric forms of α-tocopherol (*SRR-*, *SSR-*, *SRS-*, and *SSS*-α-tocopherol), also found in fortified foods and supplements.

[e] As niacin equivalents (NE). 1 mg of niacin = 60 mg of tryptophan; 0–6 months = preformed niacin (not NE).

[f] As dietary folate equivalents (DFE). 1 DFE = 1 µg food folate = 0.6 µg of folic acid from fortified food or as a supplement consumed with food = 0.5 µg of a supplement taken on an empty stomach.

[g] Although AIs have been set for choline, there are few data to assess whether a dietary supply of choline is needed at all stages of the life cycle, and it may be that the choline requirement can be met by endogenous synthesis at some of these stages.

[h] Because 10 to 30 percent of older people may malabsorb food-bound B₁₂, it is advisable for those older than 50 years to meet their RDA mainly by consuming foods fortified with B₁₂ or a supplement containing B₁₂.

[i] In view of evidence linking folate intake with neural tube defects in the fetus, it is recommended that all women capable of becoming pregnant consume 400 µg from supplements or fortified foods in addition to intake of food folate from a varied diet.

[j] It is assumed that women will continue consuming 400 µg from supplements or fortified food until their pregnancy is confirmed and they enter prenatal care, which ordinarily occurs after the end of the periconceptional period—the critical time for formation of the neural tube.

Dietary Reference Intakes (DRIs): Recommended Intakes for Individuals, Elements
Food and Nutrition Board, Institute of Medicine, National Academies

Life Stage Group	Calcium (mg/d)	Chromium (μg/d)	Copper (μg/d)	Fluoride (mg/d)	Iodine (μg/d)	Iron (mg/d)	Magnesium (mg/d)	Manganese (mg/d)	Molybdenum (μg/d)	Phosphorus (mg/d)	Selenium (μg/d)	Zinc (mg/d)	Potassium (g/d)	Sodium (g/d)	Chloride (g/d)
Infants															
0–6 mo	210*	0.2*	200*	0.01*	110*	0.27*	30*	0.003*	2*	100*	15*	2*	0.4*	0.12*	0.18*
7–12 mo	270*	5.5*	220*	0.5*	130*	11	75*	0.6*	3*	275*	20*	3	0.7*	0.37*	0.57*
Children															
1–3 y	500*	11*	340	0.7*	90	7	80	1.2*	17	460	20	3	3.0*	1.0*	1.5*
4–8 y	800*	15*	440	1*	90	10	130	1.5*	22	500	30	5	3.8*	1.2*	1.9*
Males															
9–13 y	1,300*	25*	700	2*	120	8	240	1.9*	34	1,250	40	8	4.5*	1.5*	2.3*
14–18 y	1,300*	35*	890	3*	150	11	410	2.2*	43	1,250	55	11	4.7*	1.5*	2.3*
19–30 y	1,000*	35*	900	4*	150	8	400	2.3*	45	700	55	11	4.7*	1.5*	2.3*
31–50 y	1,000*	35*	900	4*	150	8	420	2.3*	45	700	55	11	4.7*	1.5*	2.3*
51–70 y	1,200*	30*	900	4*	150	8	420	2.3*	45	700	55	11	4.7*	1.3*	2.0*
>70 y	1,200*	30*	900	4*	150	8	420	2.3*	45	700	55	11	4.7*	1.2*	1.8*
Females															
9–13 y	1,300*	21*	700	2*	120	8	240	1.6*	34	1,250	40	8	4.5*	1.5*	2.3*
14–18 y	1,300*	24*	890	3*	150	15	360	1.6*	43	1,250	55	9	4.7*	1.5*	2.3*
19–30 y	1,000*	25*	900	3*	150	18	310	1.8*	45	700	55	8	4.7*	1.5*	2.3*
31–50 y	1,000*	25*	900	3*	150	18	320	1.8*	45	700	55	8	4.7*	1.5*	2.3*
51–70 y	1,200*	20*	900	3*	150	8	320	1.8*	45	700	55	8	4.7*	1.3*	2.0*
>70 y	1,200*	20*	900	3*	150	8	320	1.8*	45	700	55	8	4.7*	1.2*	1.8*
Pregnancy															
14–18 y	1,300*	29*	1,000	3*	220	27	400	2.0*	50	1,250	60	12	4.7*	1.5*	2.3*
19–30 y	1,000*	30*	1,000	3*	220	27	350	2.0*	50	700	60	11	4.7*	1.5*	2.3*
31–50 y	1,000*	30*	1,000	3*	220	27	360	2.0*	50	700	60	11	4.7*	1.5*	2.3*
Lactation															
14–18 y	1,300*	44*	1,300	3*	290	10	360	2.6*	50	1,250	70	13	5.1*	1.5*	2.3*
19–30 y	1,000*	45*	1,300	3*	290	9	310	2.6*	50	700	70	12	5.1*	1.5*	2.3*
31–50 y	1,000*	45*	1,300	3*	290	9	320	2.6*	50	700	70	12	5.1*	1.5*	2.3*

NOTE: This table presents Recommended Dietary Allowances (RDAs) in **bold type** and Adequate Intakes (AIs) in ordinary type followed by an asterisk (*). RDAs and AIs may both be used as goals for individual intake. RDAs are set to meet the needs of almost all (97 to 98 percent) individuals in a group. For healthy breastfed infants, the AI is the mean intake. The AI for other life stage and gender groups is believed to cover needs of all individuals in the group, but lack of data or uncertainty in the data prevent being able to specify with confidence the percentage of individuals covered by this intake.

SOURCES: *Dietary Reference Intakes for Calcium, Phosphorous, Magnesium, Vitamin D, and Fluoride* (1997); *Dietary Reference Intakes for Thiamin, Riboflavin, Niacin, Vitamin B₆, Folate, Vitamin B₁₂, Pantothenic Acid, Biotin, and Choline* (1998); *Dietary Reference Intakes for Vitamin C, Vitamin E, Selenium, and Carotenoids* (2000); *Dietary Reference Intakes for Vitamin A, Vitamin K, Arsenic, Boron, Chromium, Copper, Iodine, Iron, Manganese, Molybdenum, Nickel, Silicon, Vanadium, and Zinc* (2001); and *Dietary Reference Intakes for Water, Potassium, Sodium, Chloride, and Sulfate* (2004). These reports may be accessed via http://www.nap.edu.

Copyright 2004 by the National Academy of Sciences. All rights reserved.

Dietary Reference Intakes (DRIs): Tolerable Upper Intake Levels (UL[a]), Vitamins
Food and Nutrition Board, Institute of Medicine, National Academies

Life Stage Group	Vitamin A (μg/d)[b]	Vitamin C (mg/d)	Vitamin D (μg/d)	Vitamin E (mg/d)[c,d]	Vitamin K	Thiamin	Riboflavin	Niacin (mg/d)[d]	Vitamin B6 (mg/d)	Folate (μg/d)[d]	Vitamin B12	Pantothenic Acid	Biotin	Choline (g/d)	Carotenoids[e]
Infants															
0–6 mo	600	ND[f]	25	ND	ND	ND	ND	ND	ND	ND	ND	ND	ND	ND	ND
7–12 mo	600	ND	25	ND	ND	ND	ND	ND	ND	ND	ND	ND	ND	ND	ND
Children															
1–3 y	600	400	50	200	ND	ND	ND	10	30	300	ND	ND	ND	1.0	ND
4–8 y	900	650	50	300	ND	ND	ND	15	40	400	ND	ND	ND	1.0	ND
Males, Females															
9–13 y	1,700	1,200	50	600	ND	ND	ND	20	60	600	ND	ND	ND	2.0	ND
14–18 y	2,800	1,800	50	800	ND	ND	ND	30	80	800	ND	ND	ND	3.0	ND
19–70 y	3,000	2,000	50	1,000	ND	ND	ND	35	100	1,000	ND	ND	ND	3.5	ND
>70 y	3,000	2,000	50	1,000	ND	ND	ND	35	100	1,000	ND	ND	ND	3.5	ND
Pregnancy															
14–18 y	2,800	1,800	50	800	ND	ND	ND	30	80	800	ND	ND	ND	3.0	ND
19–50 y	3,000	2,000	50	1,000	ND	ND	ND	35	100	1,000	ND	ND	ND	3.5	ND
Lactation															
14–18 y	2,800	1,800	50	800	ND	ND	ND	30	80	800	ND	ND	ND	3.0	ND
19–50 y	3,000	2,000	50	1,000	ND	ND	ND	35	100	1,000	ND	ND	ND	3.5	ND

[a] UL = The maximum level of daily nutrient intake that is likely to pose no risk of adverse effects. Unless otherwise specified, the UL represents total intake from food, water, and supplements. Due to lack of suitable data, ULs could not be established for vitamin K, thiamin, riboflavin, vitamin B12, pantothenic acid, biotin, carotenoids. In the absence of ULs, extra caution may be warranted in consuming levels above recommended intakes.

[b] As preformed vitamin A only.

[c] As α-tocopherol; applies to any form of supplemental α-tocopherol.

[d] The ULs for vitamin E, niacin, and folate apply to synthetic forms obtained from supplements, fortified foods, or a combination of the two.

[e] β-Carotene supplements are advised only to serve as a provitamin A source for individuals at risk of vitamin A deficiency.

[f] ND = Not determinable due to lack of data of adverse effects in this age group and concern with regard to lack of ability to handle excess amounts. Source of intake should be from food only to prevent high levels of intake.

SOURCES: *Dietary Reference Intakes for Calcium, Phosphorous, Magnesium, Vitamin D, and Fluoride* (1997); *Dietary Reference Intakes for Thiamin, Riboflavin, Niacin, Vitamin B6, Folate, Vitamin B12, Pantothenic Acid, Biotin, and Choline* (1998); *Dietary Reference Intakes for Vitamin C, Vitamin E, Selenium, and Carotenoids* (2000); and *Dietary Reference Intakes for Vitamin A, Vitamin K, Arsenic, Boron, Chromium, Copper, Iodine, Iron, Manganese, Molybdenum, Nickel, Silicon, Vanadium, and Zinc* (2001). These reports may be accessed via http://www.nap.edu.

Dietary Reference Intakes (DRIs): Tolerable Upper Intake Levels (UL[a]), Elements
Food and Nutrition Board, Institute of Medicine, National Academies

Life Stage Group	Arsenic[b]	Boron (mg/d)	Calcium (g/d)	Chromium	Copper (µg/d)	Fluoride (mg/d)	Iodine (µg/d)	Iron (mg/d)	Magnesium (mg/d)[c]	Manganese (mg/d)	Molybdenum (µg/d)	Nickel (mg/d)	Phosphorus (g/d)	Potassium	Selenium (µg/d)	Silicon[d]	Sulfate	Vanadium (mg/d)[e]	Zinc (mg/d)	Sodium (g/d)	Chloride (g/d)
Infants																					
0–6 mo	ND[f]	ND	ND	ND	ND	0.7	ND	40	ND	ND	ND	ND	ND	ND	45	ND	ND	ND	4	ND	ND
7–12 mo	ND	ND	ND	ND	ND	0.9	ND	40	ND	ND	ND	ND	ND	ND	60	ND	ND	ND	5	ND	ND
Children																					
1–3 y	ND	3	2.5	ND	1,000	1.3	200	40	65	2	300	0.2	3	ND	90	ND	ND	ND	7	1.5	2.3
4–8 y	ND	6	2.5	ND	3,000	2.2	300	40	110	3	600	0.3	3	ND	150	ND	ND	ND	12	1.9	2.9
Males,																					
Females																					
9–13 y	ND	11	2.5	ND	5,000	10	600	40	350	6	1,100	0.6	4	ND	280	ND	ND	ND	23	2.2	3.4
14–18 y	ND	17	2.5	ND	8,000	10	900	45	350	9	1,700	1.0	4	ND	400	ND	ND	ND	34	2.3	3.6
19–70 y	ND	20	2.5	ND	10,000	10	1,100	45	350	11	2,000	1.0	4	ND	400	ND	ND	1.8	40	2.3	3.6
>70 y	ND	20	2.5	ND	10,000	10	1,100	45	350	11	2,000	1.0	3	ND	400	ND	ND	1.8	40	2.3	3.6
Pregnancy																					
14–18 y	ND	17	2.5	ND	8,000	10	900	45	350	9	1,700	1.0	3.5	ND	400	ND	ND	ND	34	2.3	3.6
19–50 y	ND	20	2.5	ND	10,000	10	1,100	45	350	11	2,000	1.0	3.5	ND	400	ND	ND	ND	40	2.3	3.6
Lactation																					
14–18 y	ND	17	2.5	ND	8,000	10	900	45	350	9	1,700	1.0	4	ND	400	ND	ND	ND	34	2.3	3.6
19–50 y	ND	20	2.5	ND	10,000	10	1,100	45	350	11	2,000	1.0	4	ND	400	ND	ND	ND	40	2.3	3.6

[a] UL = The maximum level of daily nutrient intake that is likely to pose no risk of adverse effects. Unless otherwise specified, the UL represents total intake from food, water, and supplements. Due to lack of suitable data, ULs could not be established for arsenic, chromium, silicon, potassium, and sulfate. In the absence of ULs, extra caution may be warranted in consuming levels above recommended intakes.

[b] Although the UL was not determined for arsenic, there is no justification for adding arsenic to food or supplements.

[c] The ULs for magnesium represent intake from a pharmacological agent only and do not include intake from food and water.

[d] Although silicon has not been shown to cause adverse effects in humans, there is no justification for adding silicon to supplements.

[e] Although vanadium in food has not been shown to cause adverse effects in humans, there is no justification for adding vanadium to food and vanadium supplements should be used with caution. The UL is based on adverse effects in laboratory animals and this data could be used to set a UL for adults but not children and adolescents.

[f] ND = Not determinable due to lack of data of adverse effects in this age group and concern with regard to lack of ability to handle excess amounts. Source of intake should be from food only to prevent high levels of intake.

SOURCES: *Dietary Reference Intakes for Calcium, Phosphorous, Magnesium, Vitamin D, and Fluoride* (1997); *Dietary Reference Intakes for Thiamin, Riboflavin, Niacin, Vitamin B[6], Folate, Vitamin B[12], Pantothenic Acid, Biotin, and Choline* (1998); *Dietary Reference Intakes for Vitamin C, Vitamin E, Selenium, and Carotenoids* (2000); *Dietary Reference Intakes for Vitamin A, Vitamin K, Arsenic, Boron, Chromium, Copper, Iodine, Iron, Manganese, Molybdenum, Nickel, Silicon, Vanadium, and Zinc* (2001); and *Dietary Reference Intakes for Water, Potassium, Sodium, Chloride, and Sulfate* (2004). These reports may be accessed via http://www.nap.edu.

Dietary Reference Intakes (DRIs): Estimated Energy Requirements (EER) for Men and Women 30 Years of Age[a]

Food and Nutrition Board, Institute of Medicine, National Academies

Height (m [in])	PAL[b]	Weight for BMI[c] of 18.5 kg/m^2 (kg [lb])	Weight for BMI of 24.99 kg/m^2 (kg [lb])	EER, Men[d] (kcal/day) BMI of 18.5 kg/m^2	BMI of 24.99 kg/m^2	EER, Women[d] (kcal/day) BMI of 18.5 kg/m^2	BMI of 24.99 kg/m^2
1.50 (59)	Sedentary	41.6 (92)	56.2 (124)	1,848	2,080	1,625	1,762
	Low active			2,009	2,267	1,803	1,956
	Active			2,215	2,506	2,025	2,198
	Very active			2,554	2,898	2,291	2,489
1.65 (65)	Sedentary	50.4 (111)	68.0 (150)	2,068	2,349	1,816	1,982
	Low active			2,254	2,566	2,016	2,202
	Active			2,490	2,842	2,267	2,477
	Very active			2,880	3,296	2,567	2,807
1.80 (71)	Sedentary	59.9 (132)	81.0 (178)	2,301	2,635	2,015	2,211
	Low active			2,513	2,884	2,239	2,459
	Active			2,782	3,200	2,519	2,769
	Very active			3,225	3,720	2,855	3,141

[a] For each year below 30, add 7 kcal/day for women and 10 kcal/day for men. For each year above 30, subtract 7 kcal/day for women and 10 kcal/day for men.

[b] PAL = physical activity level.

[c] BMI = body mass index.

[d] Derived from the following regression equations based on doubly labeled water data:

   Adult man: $EER = 662 - 9.53 \times age\ (y) + PA \times (15.91 \times wt\ [kg] + 539.6 \times ht\ [m])$

   Adult woman: $EER = 354 - 6.91 \times age\ (y) + PA \times (9.36 \times wt\ [kg] + 726 \times ht\ [m])$

Where PA refers to coefficient for PAL

PAL = total energy expenditure + basal energy expenditure

   PA = 1.0 if PAL ≥ 1.0 < 1.4 (sedentary)

   PA = 1.12 if PAL ≥ 1.4 < 1.6 (low active)

   PA = 1.27 if PAL ≥ 1.6 < 1.9 (active)

   PA = 1.45 if PAL ≥ 1.9 < 2.5 (very active)

Dietary Reference Intakes (DRIs): Acceptable Macronutrient Distribution Ranges

Food and Nutrition Board, Institute of Medicine, National Academies

Macronutrient	Range (percent of energy) Children, 1–3 y	Children, 4–18 y	Adults
Fat	30–40	25–35	20–35
n-6 polyunsaturated fatty acids[a] (linoleic acid)	5–10	5–10	5–10
n-3 polyunsaturated fatty acids[a] (α-linolenic acid)	0.6–1.2	0.6–1.2	0.6–1.2
Carbohydrate	45–65	45–65	45–65
Protein	5–20	10–30	10–35

[a] Approximately 10% of the total can come from longer-chain n-3 or n-6 fatty acids.

SOURCE: *Dietary Reference Intakes for Energy, Carbohydrate, Fiber, Fat, Fatty Acids, Cholesterol, Protein, and Amino Acids* (2002).

Dietary Reference Intakes (DRIs): Recommended Intakes for Individuals, Macronutrients
Food and Nutrition Board, Institute of Medicine, National Academies

Life Stage Group	Total Water[a] (L/d)	Carbohydrate (g/d)	Total Fiber (g/d)	Fat (g/d)	Linoleic Acid (g/d)	⊠-Linolenic Acid (g/d)	Protein[b] (g/d)
Infants							
0–6 mo	0.7*	60*	ND	31*	4.4*	0.5*	9.1*
7–12 mo	0.8*	95*	ND	30*	4.6*	0.5*	**11.0**[c]
Children							
1–3 y	1.3*	**130**	19*	ND	7*	0.7*	**13**
4–8 y	1.7*	**130**	25*	ND	10*	0.9*	**19**
Males							
9–13 y	2.4*	**130**	31*	ND	12*	1.2*	**34**
14–18 y	3.3*	**130**	38*	ND	16*	1.6*	**52**
19–30 y	3.7*	**130**	38*	ND	17*	1.6*	**56**
31–50 y	3.7*	**130**	38*	ND	17*	1.6*	**56**
51–70 y	3.7*	**130**	30*	ND	14*	1.6*	**56**
> 70 y	3.7*	**130**	30*	ND	14*	1.6*	**56**
Females							
9–13 y	2.1*	**130**	26*	ND	10*	1.0*	**34**
14–18 y	2.3*	**130**	26*	ND	11*	1.1*	**46**
19–30 y	2.7*	**130**	25*	ND	12*	1.1*	**46**
31–50 y	2.7*	**130**	25*	ND	12*	1.1*	**46**
51–70 y	2.7*	**130**	21*	ND	11*	1.1*	**46**
> 70 y	2.7*	**130**	21*	ND	11*	1.1*	**46**
Pregnancy							
14–18 y	3.0*	**175**	28*	ND	13*	1.4*	**71**
19–30 y	3.0*	**175**	28*	ND	13*	1.4*	**71**
31–50 y	3.0*	**175**	28*	ND	13*	1.4*	**71**
Lactation							
14–18 y	3.8*	**210**	29*	ND	13*	1.3*	**71**
19–30 y	3.8*	**210**	29*	ND	13*	1.3*	**71**
31–50 y	3.8*	**210**	29*	ND	13*	1.3*	**71**

NOTE: This table presents Recommended Dietary Allowances (RDAs) in **bold** type and Adequate Intakes (AIs) in ordinary type followed by an asterisk (*). RDAs and AIs may both be used as goals for individual intake. RDAs are set to meet the needs of almost all (97 to 98 percent) individuals in a group. For healthy infants fed human milk, the AI is the mean intake. The AI for other life stage and gender groups is believed to cover the needs of all individuals in the group, but lack of data or uncertainty in the data prevent being able to specify with confidence the percentage of individuals covered by this intake.
[a] *Total* water includes all water contained in food, beverages, and drinking water.
[b] Based on 0.8 g/kg body weight for the reference body weight.
[c] Change from 13.5 in prepublication copy due to calculation error.

Dietary Reference Intakes (DRIs): Additional Macronutrient Recommendations
Food and Nutrition Board, Institute of Medicine, National Academies

Macronutrient	Recommendation
Dietary cholesterol	As low as possible while consuming a nutritionally adequate diet
Trans fatty acids	As low as possible while consuming a nutritionally adequate diet
Saturated fatty acids	As low as possible while consuming a nutritionally adequate diet
Added sugars	Limit to no more than 25% of total energy

SOURCE: *Dietary Reference Intakes for Energy, Carbohydrate, Fiber, Fat, Fatty Acids, Cholesterol, Protein, and Amino Acids* (2002).

Dietary Reference Intakes (DRIs): Estimated Average Requirements for Groups

Food and Nutrition Board, Institute of Medicine, National Academies

Life Stage Group	CHO (g/d)	Protein (g/d)[a]	Vit A (μg/d)[b]	Vit C (mg/d)	Vit E (mg/d)[c]	Thiamin (mg/d)	Riboflavin (mg/d)	Niacin (mg/d)[d]	Vit B6 (mg/d)	Folate (μg/d)[b]	Vit B12 (μg/d)	Copper (μg/d)	Iodine (μg/d)	Iron (mg/d)	Magnesium (mg/d)	Molybdenum (μg/d)	Phosphorus (mg/d)	Selenium (μg/d)	Zinc (mg/d)
Infants																			
7–12 mo		9*												6.9					2.5
Children																			
1–3 y	100	11	210	13	5	0.4	0.4	5	0.4	120	0.7	260	65	3.0	65	13	380	17	2.5
4–8 y	100	15	275	22	6	0.5	0.5	6	0.5	160	1.0	340	65	4.1	110	17	405	23	4.0
Males																			
9–13 y	100	27	445	39	9	0.7	0.8	9	0.8	250	1.5	540	73	5.9	200	26	1,055	35	7.0
14–18 y	100	44	630	63	12	1.0	1.1	12	1.1	330	2.0	685	95	7.7	340	33	1,055	45	8.5
19–30 y	100	46	625	75	12	1.0	1.1	12	1.1	320	2.0	700	95	6	330	34	580	45	9.4
31–50 y	100	46	625	75	12	1.0	1.1	12	1.1	320	2.0	700	95	6	350	34	580	45	9.4
51–70 y	100	46	625	75	12	1.0	1.1	12	1.4	320	2.0	700	95	6	350	34	580	45	9.4
>70 y	100	46	625	75	12	1.0	1.1	12	1.4	320	2.0	700	95	6	350	34	580	45	9.4
Females																			
9–13 y	100	28	420	39	9	0.7	0.8	9	0.8	250	1.5	540	73	5.7	200	26	1,055	35	7.0
14–18 y	100	38	485	56	12	0.9	0.9	11	1.0	330	2.0	685	95	7.9	300	33	1,055	45	7.3
19–30 y	100	38	500	60	12	0.9	0.9	11	1.1	320	2.0	700	95	8.1	255	34	580	45	6.8
31–50 y	100	38	500	60	12	0.9	0.9	11	1.1	320	2.0	700	95	8.1	265	34	580	45	6.8
51–70 y	100	38	500	60	12	0.9	0.9	11	1.3	320	2.0	700	95	5	265	34	580	45	6.8
>70 y	100	38	500	60	12	0.9	0.9	11	1.3	320	2.0	700	95	5	265	34	580	45	6.8
Pregnancy																			
14–18 y	135	50	530	66	12	1.2	1.2	14	1.6	520	2.2	785	160	23	335	40	1,055	49	10.5
19–30 y	135	50	550	70	12	1.2	1.2	14	1.6	520	2.2	800	160	22	290	40	580	49	9.5
31–50 y	135	50	550	70	12	1.2	1.2	14	1.6	520	2.2	800	160	22	300	40	580	49	9.5
Lactation																			
14–18 y	160	60	885	96	16	1.2	1.3	13	1.7	450	2.4	985	209	7	300	35	1,055	59	10.9
19–30 y	160	60	900	100	16	1.2	1.3	13	1.7	450	2.4	1,000	209	6.5	255	36	580	59	10.4
31–50 y	160	60	900	100	16	1.2	1.3	13	1.7	450	2.4	1,000	209	6.5	265	36	580	59	10.4

NOTE: This table presents Estimated Average Requirements (EARs), which serve two purposes: for assessing adequacy of population intakes, and as the basis for calculating Recommended Dietary Allowances (RDAs) for individuals for those nutrients. EARs have not been established for vitamin D, vitamin K, pantothenic acid, biotin, choline, calcium, chromium, fluoride, manganese, or other nutrients not yet evaluated via the DRI process.

[a] For individual at reference weight (Table 1-1). *indicates change from prepublication copy due to calculation error.

[b] As retinol activity equivalents (RAEs). 1 RAE = 1 μg retinol, 12 μg β-carotene, 24 μg α-carotene, or 24 μg β-cryptoxanthin. The RAE for dietary provitamin A carotenoids is two-fold greater than retinol equivalents (RE), whereas the RAE for preformed vitamin A is the same as RE.

[c] As α-tocopherol. α-Tocopherol includes RRR-α-tocopherol, the only form of α-tocopherol that occurs naturally in foods, and the 2R-stereoisomeric forms of α-tocopherol (RRR-, RSR-, RRS-, and RSS-α-tocopherol) that occur in fortified foods and supplements. It does not include the 2S-stereoisomeric forms of α-tocopherol (SRR-, SSR-, SRS-, and SSS-α-tocopherol), also found in fortified foods and supplements.

[d] As niacin equivalents (NE). 1 mg of niacin = 60 mg of tryptophan.

[e] As dietary folate equivalents (DFE). 1 DFE = 1 μg food folate = 0.6 μg of folic acid from fortified food or as a supplement consumed with food = 0.5 μg of a supplement taken on an empty stomach.

SOURCES: *Dietary Reference Intakes for Calcium, Phosphorous, Magnesium, Vitamin D, and Fluoride* (1997); *Dietary Reference Intakes for Thiamin, Riboflavin, Niacin, Vitamin B₆, Folate, Vitamin B₁₂, Pantothenic Acid, Biotin, and Choline* (1998); *Dietary Reference Intakes for Vitamin C, Vitamin E, Selenium, and Carotenoids* (2000); *Dietary Reference Intakes for Vitamin A, Vitamin K, Arsenic, Boron, Chromium, Copper, Iodine, Iron, Manganese, Molybdenum, Nickel, Silicon, Vanadium, and Zinc* (2001), and *Dietary Reference Intakes for Energy, Carbohydrate, Fiber, Fat, Fatty Acids, Cholesterol, Protein, and Amino Acids* (2002). These reports may be accessed via www.nap.edu.

Resources

Appendix

D

To support you on your journey further along the plant-based path, I've compiled this appendix full of many helpful resources to make it easier for you to connect with fellow plant-foodists, continue learning, buy specialty food items, and find more delicious recipes.

Nutrition Information Books

Anderson, Mike. *The RAVE Diet and Lifestyle.* www.RaveDiet.com. 2004.

Barnard, Neal D. *21-Day Weight Loss Kickstart.* New York: Grand Central Life and Style, 2011.

———. *Breaking the Food Seduction.* New York: St. Martin's Griffin, 2003.

———. *Dr. Neal Barnard's Program for Reversing Diabetes.* New York: Rodale, 2007.

Bennett, Beverly Lynn, and Ray Sammartano. *The Complete Idiot's Guide to Vegan Living.* Indianapolis: Alpha Books, 2005.

Brazier, Brendan. *Thrive: The Vegan Nutrition Guide to Optimal Performance in Sports and Life.* Philadelphia: Da Capo Press, 2007.

Campbell, T. Colin, and T. M. Campbell. *The China Study.* Dallas: Benbella Books, 2006.

Davis, Brenda, and Vesanto Melina. *Becoming Raw.* Summertown, TN: Book Publishing Company, 2010.

———. *Becoming Vegan.* Summertown, TN: Book Publishing Company, 2000.

Esselstyn, Caldwell B. *Prevent and Reverse Heart Disease*. New York: Penguin Group, 2007.

Esselstyn, Rip. *The Engine 2 Diet*. New York: Wellness Central, 2009.

Freedman, Rory, and K. Barnouin. *Skinny Bitch*. Philadelphia: Running Press, 2005.

Fuhrman, Joel. *Disease-Proof Your Child*. New York: St. Martin's Griffin, 2005.

———. *Eat for Health*. Flemington, NJ: Gift of Health Press, 2008.

———. *Eat to Live*. New York: Little, Brown and Company, 2011.

Kessler, David. *The End of Overeating*. Emmaus: Rodale, 2010.

Lisle, Doug J., and A. Goldhamer. *The Pleasure Trap*. Summertown, TN: Healthy Living, 2003.

McDougall, John A. *Dr. McDougall's Digestive Tune-Up*. Summertown, TN: Healthy Living, 2006.

———. *The Starch Solution*. Emmaus: Rodale, 2012.

Robbins, John. *Healthy at 100*. New York: Ballantine Books, 2007.

———. *The Food Revolution*. Boston: Conari Press, 2010.

Stepaniak, Jo. *The Vegan Sourcebook*. New York: McGraw Hill, 2000.

Plant-Based Cookbooks

Barnard, Tanya, and S. Kramer. *How It All Vegan*. Vancouver: Arsenal Pulp Press, 1999.

———. *The Garden of Vegan*. Vancouver: Arsenal Pulp Press, 2002.

Bennett, Beverly Lynn, and Ray Sammartano. *The Complete Idiot's Guide to Vegan Cooking*. Indianapolis: Alpha Books, 2008.

Burton, Dreena. *Eat, Drink and Be Vegan*. Vancouver: Arsenal Pulp Press, 2007.

Chef AJ. *Unprocessed*. Los Angeles: Hail to the Kale Publishing, 2011.

Hever, Julieanna, and Beverly Lynn Bennett. *The Complete Idiot's Guide to Gluten-Free Vegan Cooking*. Indianapolis: Alpha Books, 2011.

Kramer, Sarah. *Vegan A Go-Go*. Vancouver: Arsenal Pulp Press, 2008.

Moskowitz, Isa C., and T. H. Romero. *Veganomicon: The Ultimate Vegan Cookbook*. New York: Marlowe and Company, 2007.

Patrick-Goudreau, C. *Color Me Vegan*. Beverly, MA: Fair Winds Press, 2010.

————. *The Vegan Table*. Beverly, MA: Fair Winds Press, 2009.

Robertson, Robin. *1,000 Vegan Recipes*. Hoboken: John Wiley and Sons, 2009.

————. *Vegan on the Cheap*. Hoboken: John Wiley and Sons, 2010.

Stepaniak, Jo. *The Ultimate Uncheese Cookbook, 10th Edition*. Summertown, TN: Book Publishing Company, 2003.

Nutrition and Health Information, Recipes, and Support

American College of Lifestyle Medicine
www.lifestylemedicine.org

American Dietetic Associations' Vegetarian Group
www.vegetariannutrition.net

Brenda Davis, R.D.
www.brendadavisrd.com

Chef AJ
www.chefajshealthykitchen.com

Chef Beverly Lynn Bennett
www.veganchef.com

Coronary Health Improvement Project
www.chiphealth.com

Dr. Joel Fuhrman
www.drfuhrman.com

Dr. McDougall's Health and Medical Center
www.drmcdougall.com

EarthSave, International
www.earthsave.org

Engine 2 Diet
www.engine2diet.com

Fatfree Vegan Recipes
www.fatfreevegan.com

Forks Over Knives
www.plantbaseddiet.com

HappyCow (for plant-based dining options)
www.happycow.net

John Robbins
www.johnrobbins.info

Physicians Committee for Responsible Medicine (PCRM)
www.pcrm.org

Plant-Based Dietitian
www.plantbaseddietitian.com
toyourhealthnutrition.blogspot.com

T. Colin Campbell Foundation
www.tcolincampbell.org

TrueNorth Health Center
www.healthpromoting.com

Vegetarian Resource Group
www.vrg.org

Vegetarians in Paradise
www.vegparadise.com

VegNews **magazine**
www.vegnews.com

VegSource
www.vegsource.com

Where to Order Food Products

Cosmo's Vegan Shoppe
www.cosmosveganshoppe.com

Dragünara (spices and sauces)
www.dragunara.com

Organics Are for Everyone (date paste)
www.organicsareforeveryone.com

SunSpire (grain-sweetened chocolate chips)
www.sunspire.com

Vegan Essentials
www.veganessentials.com

Vitacost
www.vitacost.com

Index